LOGIC IN MEDICINE

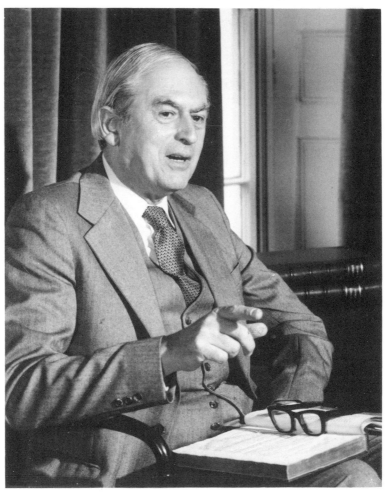

Sir Peter Medawar, to whom this book is dedicated.

LOGIC IN MEDICINE

Edited by
CALBERT I PHILLIPS, MD, PHD
Professor of Ophthalmology
University of Edinburgh

Articles from the *British Medical Journal*
Published by the British Medical Journal
Tavistock Square, London WC1H 9JR

The painting on the front cover, Head of a Surgeon, is by John Smalley.

ISBN 0 7279 0217 2

Typeset by Bedford Typesetters Ltd, Bedford, and printed by the University Press, Belfast

Contents

INTRODUCTION

CALBERT I PHILLIPS

All medical students and practitioners have an interest in the thought processes that lead to diagnosis. Although clinical medicine is often concerned with examples of diagnostic logic, a general philosophy is seldom discussed. The individual infers his own generalisations from particular cases. An intuitive approach based on experience usually serves remarkably well. Implicit in most systems is the law of economy of hypotheses (William of Occam's razor), with due respect to the numerous exceptions. Concepts of probability and the null hypothesis and their application from statistics make a useful contribution.

The major aim of this series is to present and discuss a coherent system of "diagnostic logic," which is the subject of the third paper by Professor Fergus Macartney. He starts by questioning the need for diagnosis at all and concludes that complete precision is often unnecessary. He shows with examples the importance of Bayes's theorem, granting some limitations. This concept probably forms the basis for the logic of diagnosis. "Pattern recognition" oversimplifies it. The merits of the hypotheticodeductive approach are discussed. Aesthetic appeal is offered as a sufficient reason for logical parsimony, but economic parsimony (given the scarcity of resources) is a compelling reason for abandoning the traditional blunderbuss method of diagnosis.

Dr Knill-Jones, dealing with decision making, discusses the use of weighting, modified to take account of interdependence of symptoms and signs, and shows how this formulation of Bayes's theorem is related to the more familiar landmarks of sensitivity, specificity, and relative risk.

There may be some truth in the charge (easily defended) that medical education is too narrowly vocational and that our students have too little opportunity to benefit from the wider academic environment of the universities (even in basic medical science). Surely diagnostic logic must be based on the same principles as logic in general?

Two members of the department of philosophy in the University of Edinburgh have provided a more general perspective for our applied medical systems. Granted that making a diagnosis is a rather different activity from establishing a scientific theory, the evolution of scientific method is important for both. The first paper, by Dr Briskman, shows how the philosophy of empirical science has achieved its present supremacy. Its adventures of ideas have progressed from preinductivism to Baconian induction; but that carried the seeds of its own destruction, according to Hume's criticisms. Karl Popper's more constructive use of unbelief is advocated in the principle of refutability or falsifiability, a necessary property of any theory before it can achieve the status of empirical science. Professor Macartney also discusses the interrelationship between the application of the Popper approach and the hypotheticodeductive model.

Dr Slaney's remit is to provide an impression of the present state of the very large subject of logic (or the abstract theory of theories), with reference where possible to a medical content. We discover that his dynamic and open ended subject is tentative and exploratory, like all science, and that its various systems pay the price of selectivity to achieve increased precision. Ultimately these systems depend on analogy, which, by its nature, can never provide a completely secure foundation. He explores various aspects of inference. As in the third and fourth articles, the importance of computer technology and artificially intelligent expert systems is clear. He introduces two varieties of unorthodox logic with potential practical application to our discipline. Because medicine has to deal with imprecise descriptions whose truth is a matter of degree, "fuzzy logic" applies well to it; and because automated reasoning seems to be most efficient when using logic no stronger than is necessary, "relevant logic" may be of value in many applications of expert systems.

It is easier to indulge perfectionism in abstract ideas than in their practical application. Assumptions we take for granted are the constraints of various laws of nature as we perceive them—and as we modify them progressively as empirical science advances. Our theories have to be applied in an economic environment with scarce resources, and in a social and an ethical environment demanding high standards. The practical necessity for economic parsimony supports (explains?) our intuitive attraction towards logical parsimony. We can and do easily exaggerate the importance of a conflict of interest between the individual and the community.

Professor Maynard shows that many of our medical (and other) problems in Britain come from our low ranking in the prosperity table. The more prosperous a country, the higher the proportion of its gross national product it spends on health care. Even in a rich country, however, demand and need for health care outstrip available resources. Systematic identification and analysis of the imposed choices and rationing are the essence of the logic of economics. Two important terms are explained. The opportunity cost of any given choice is the value of the best option that is foregone. The margin is the increment added to costs (or outcomes) by one unit change in the level of activity. A law of diminishing returns applies when very expensive and distressful treatment prolongs existence: mere survival is no longer the only criterion for success in treatment, hence the notion of the "quality adjusted life year." John Maynard Keynes said "Practical men . . . are usually slaves of some defunct economist." Whatever our prejudices from whatever sources, we can probably agree with Professor Maynard when he asserts that inefficiency is unethical and that to avoid the unethical it is essential to evaluate costs and outcomes systematically.

Ethics are as all pervasive as logic and economics in medicine, although their importance is less overtly recognised. Historical contingency and wide cultural diversity may appear to lead to scepticism and moral relativism. On the contrary, Dr Thompson adduces general historical, cultural, and philosophical arguments to demonstrate the fundamental nature of the interdependent principles of respect for persons, justice, and beneficence. More positively, they inspire us to idealism. In ethics, even more than in other parts of philosophy and logic, we accept intuitively as a premise freedom of will—which is indispensable for the regulation of society.

Doctors and witchdoctors: Which doctors are which?

LARRY BRISKMAN

"Mark this, ye proud men of action," wrote the great German poet and philosopher Heinrich Heine, "Ye are nothing but unconscious instruments of the men of thought who, often in humblest seclusion, have appointed you to your inevitable task. Maximillian Robespierre was merely the hand of Jean-Jacques Rousseau. . . ."[1] This testimony to the power of ideas, even philosophical ideas, over even the most practical of men is echoed in our century by John Maynard Keynes.[2] "The ideas of economists and political philosophers," he wrote, "both when they are right and when they are wrong, are more powerful than is commonly understood. Indeed, the world is ruled by little else. Practical men, who believe themselves to be quite exempt from any intellectual influences, are usually the slaves of some defunct economist. Madmen in authority, who hear voices in the air, are distilling their frenzy from some academic scribbler of a few years back. I am sure that the power of vested interests is vastly exaggerated compared with the gradual encroachment of ideas . . . soon or late, it is ideas, not vested interests, which are dangerous for good or evil."

Members of the medical profession are not, of course, all "madmen in authority"; but they are practical men, and they do, in Western society at least, enjoy positions of considerable authority. This status is not fundamentally political, nor is it essentially economic. Rather, members of the medical profession derive whatever political and economic status (or power) they have from their recognised intellectual status. It is this that explains why economic resources in the West are directed to the practice and improvement of medicine (as opposed to the practice and improvement of, say, witchcraft); and it also explains why, for example, Western courts of law recognise qualified medical practitioners as being "expert" witnesses on many matters whereas the practitioners of faith healing or Christian Science, who

1

claim to have performed many medical miracles, are not so recognised. From what source does the medical profession derive its generally acknowledged intellectual status? More precisely, what is it that demarcates Western medical science from the claims of witchcraft, faith healing, Christian Science, and so on?

This question, or rather a generalisation of it, is one of the fundamental problems of the philosophy of science: the problem of demarcation. How can we distinguish genuine empirical science from pseudoempirical superstition or pseudoscience? In so far as members of the medical profession, and the general public, attribute to Western medical science an intellectual status superior to that of witchcraft, faith healing, and so on, they are assuming (if only implicitly) that there is some solution to this problem. Doctors who, as practical men, believe themselves to be exempt from any intellectual influences of a philosophical kind may thus turn out to be the slaves of some defunct philosopher of science. Rather than being impotent, philosophical ideas about science are at the root of medicine's social and economic influence.

The problem of demarcation

The problem of demarcation is not merely a matter of definition or of words; if it were it would be quite uninteresting. The problem is not that of trying to reach agreement on how the term "empirical science" is to be used as opposed to the terms "superstition" or "pseudoscience." Rather, the problem is basically one of explaining why, if at all, we should take the claims or theories of empirical science (and in particular those of medical science) more seriously than we do those of witchcraft, faith healing, Christian Science, or scientology.

This problem is of serious importance for medicine for the basis of Western medical practice would seem to be our scientific knowledge of diseases, their causes, and their cures. But this statement, though plausible enough, in fact rather understates the case—or many of the triumphs of medical science have nothing to do with disease (in its usual sense) at all. For example, having a hand cut off by a combine harvester is hardly a case of disease, yet we have developed microsurgical techniques to help to "cure" this affliction. Clearly these techniques depend on much more than a biological knowledge of the human body (its circulatory and nervous systems and so on). They also depend on our knowledge of physics—for example, the use of powerful optical instruments—and pharmacology, and the development of drugs clearly depends on chemical knowledge. Thus the basis of Western medical practice is almost the whole of empirical science.

If we are to explain why Western medical practice is preferable to the practices of, say, the witchdoctor we need to explain why the claims or theories of empirical science deserve to be preferred, from the point of view of truth, to those of witchcraft—that is, we need to solve the problem of demarcation. It is important to realise why this is so. If a patient suffering from a high fever comes to a doctor and the doctor, after examination, diagnoses a bacterial infection and prescribes penicillin he is making use of a considerable body of scientific knowledge. If the same patient went to a witchdoctor the techniques of examination, the diagnosis, and the prescribed cure would be very different. For example, the examination might include a study of the entrails of a live chicken; the diagnosis might be that the fever is the result of a spell; and the prescribed cure might be some sort of ritual purification or some sort of symbolic action (such as sticking pins in an effigy of the person identified as casting the spell).

Such prescribed cures are, of course, "ritual" or "symbolic" from our point of view (and, dare I say, in reality as well); but from the viewpoint of the "magic circle" of witchcraft ideas they are neither ritual nor symbolic. They are instrumental or technological. In other words, given the witchdoctor's view of the world—that is, given his theories—his techniques of examination and diagnosis and his prescribed cure are just as rational as their Western medical counterparts (in the sense of "weak rationality"[3]). But this entails (I almost said "entrails"), if we are to explain why our medical practice is preferable to the witchdoctor's, seeking the explanation in some difference between the knowledge or theories that we use and the knowledge or theories that he uses. In other words, we need to distinguish—or demarcate—genuine empirical science, which deserves to be taken seriously from the point of view of truth, from pseudoempirical superstitions like the theories of witchcraft, which are not so deserving.

In what way can superstitions, like the theories of witchcraft, be pseudoempirical? The answer is that such theories can seem to be supported or confirmed by empirical or observational evidence. Thus take any illness that would, if left completely untreated, spontaneously remit—for example, the common cold; or any illness whose symptoms appear only intermittently—for example, herpes; or any illness whose initial primary symptoms disappear altogether to be followed only much later by different, often more severe, symptoms —for example, syphilis. Then even if we assume that the practices of the witchdoctor have no efficacy whatsoever in curing illness these practices will *seem* to have many successes (we assume, for the sake of simplicity, that the proposed cures of the witchdoctor are not themselves injurious to health). Thus despite their superstitious character the assumptions on which the witchdoctor bases his practice can often seem to receive empirical support or confirmation. Yet in the cases described such support, or pseudosupport, is spurious. Indeed, one way of putting the problem of demarcation is precisely this: How can we distinguish between genuine empirical support (or a genuine empirical method) and spurious or pseudoempirical support (or a pseudoempirical method)?

Bacon's inductivist solution

In the British philosophical tradition the generally accepted solution to these problems stems from the inductivist philosophy of Francis Bacon. According to this view what distinguishes genuine empirical science (or support) from pseudoempirical superstition (or pseudosupport) is the use of a certain method—the inductive method. Empirical science is the product of its application, superstitious pseudoscience is not. What distinguishes the scientist (who employs induction) is that he always begins his investigation of the world without preconceived ideas: he approaches the world with an open mind and makes empirical observations in an unprejudiced manner. Only after he has collected a sufficient body of unprejudiced observations does he begin to try, using these observations, to discover their underlying causes or explanation—and this he does by the inductive method of inferring their causes or explanation from the observational evidence itself.

The method of superstition (or, as Bacon called it, the method of anticipation or speculation) is quite different from this. Here, rather than allowing our ideas to be determined by the observed facts, we *begin* with ideas—that is to say, with sheer conjectures about the causes or explanations of phenomena—and then proceed, as we saw

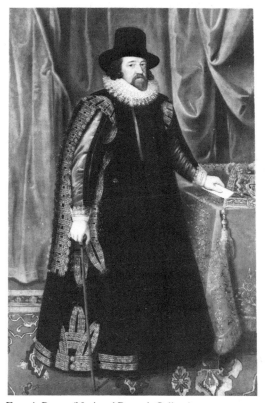

Francis Bacon (National Portrait Gallery).

was possible with the witchdoctor, to find empirical or observational evidence to support or "confirm" our preconceived ideas. Thus those who use this method do not begin with an open mind and attempt to accommodate their ideas to their observations (as does the scientist); rather, they begin with an idea and attempt to accommodate their observations to their ideas.

According to Baconian inductivism the fact that observational evidence that apparently supports a preconceived idea can be found is really neither here nor there—for it is always possible to find such support. Such apparent support is spurious or pseudosupport as it was gathered in the light of the very idea that it was supposed to support. The support that is called on in the use of the inductive method, on the other hand, is genuine or real support for here the support came before the idea and so could not possibly have been "rigged up" in the light of it. In other words, the method of anticipation, by starting with the idea to be confirmed, allows its practitioner to interpret observations made in the light of his idea as confirmatory support for his idea; but those who practise the method of induction cannot possibly do this.

The traditional solution to the problem of demarcation—the inductivist solution—amounts, then, to this: what distinguishes genuinely scientific knowledge and genuinely scientific theories from pseudoscientific superstition is the application of the inductive method of inquiry. Genuine empirical science results from its application; pseudoscientific superstition does not. As a result the theories of empirical science are genuinely supported by our observations and experiments—and thus deserve to be taken seriously from the point of view of truth—whereas those of witchcraft (and other superstitions) are not genuinely supported by the evidence—and thus are not so deserving.

Something like this inductivist solution to the problem of demarcation is, I suspect, accepted by many doctors (and, indeed, by many scientists). It is also, I suggest, accepted by most members of the general public. This acceptance is reflected in the common image of the scientist as an unprejudiced searcher after truth—one who sticks closely to the facts and does not speculate in advance of them; who does not allow his observations to be clouded by preconceived ideas; and who puts forward only those theories that can be deduced from the unprejudiced facts. This view of science was summed up by the incomparable Mr Newton (as John Locke called him): "The main business of natural philosophy [that is, of empirical science] is to argue from phenomena without feigning hypotheses, and to deduce causes from effects." It is the view of scientific method popularised by Sherlock Holmes: Conan Doyle was, after all, a medical doctor.

The above considerations are, of course, elementary (my dear Watson). Yet only 50 years after Newton's *Principia*, and some 150 years before Conan Doyle, the inductivist solution to the problem of demarcation was refuted by the great Scottish philosopher David Hume.[4] That most contemporary philosophers of science, although highly appreciative of Hume, do not recognise Hume's achievement is testimony to the lasting influence of inductivist ideas.

Hume's refutation of inductivism

Hume's refutation of the inductivist solution to the problem of demarcation rests on his discovery that the inductive method itself requires what is, given the inductivist solution, a pseudoempirical superstition. In other words, from the point of view of inductivism, empirical science, rather than being demarcated from superstition, is simply another form of superstition. For if what distinguishes or demarcates empirical science from pseudoempirical superstition is the use of the inductive method, and if Hume is right in arguing that this method itself depends on or requires the assumption of a pseudoempirical superstition, then empirical science is just a pseudo-empirical superstition and so cannot be demarcated from it. Induction, the philosopher C D Broad lamented, which was thought to be the glory of science, turns out to be the scandal of philosophy.

How did Hume show that the inductive method itself depends on a pseudoempirical superstition? To see this, return for a moment to the fundamental rules of inductive method: (*a*) start from observations, not speculations, and do not allow any preconceived ideas to prejudice

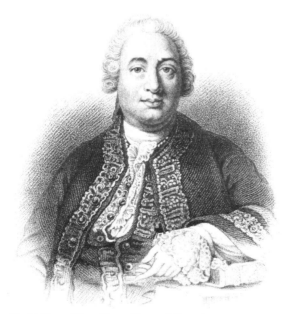

David Hume (Mary Evans Picture Library).

empirical observation; (b) after collecting a sufficient body of observations (of particular effects) infer their underlying causes or the universal laws of nature that explain them. It is quite clear from these rules, and especially from rule (b), that inductivism requires us to be able to reason from the observation of effects to their underlying causes, or from the observation of particular instances to the universal laws that explain them.

Hume's argument can now be formulated as follows: every inference, or process of reasoning, from observed effects to their underlying causes or from observed particulars to universal laws, is effectively an inference from what has been found in observation (or in "experience," as it is sometimes put) to that which is not found in observation (experience). For though the observable effects can, of course, be observed, the underlying causes cannot be observed; and though particular instances of a universal law can be observed, the universality of such a law cannot be observed. But this means that every inductive inference (from effects to causes or from particulars to universal laws) must make use of a "hidden" assumption—the assumption that observed effects are a good guide to their underlying causes or that observed particulars are good guides to universal laws. In general, the inductivist must assume that unprejudiced observation is a good guide to what lies beyond observation, or that experience is a good guide to what lies outwith it.

Now, asks Hume, does the inductivist have a right, from his own point of view, to make any such assumption? According to the inductivist solution to the problem of demarcation such an assumption should be made only if it itself can be reached in accordance with rules (a) and (b); otherwise it is merely a preconceived idea to be shunned by genuine empirical science. But it is clear, argues Hume, that it cannot be so reached. For to reach this assumption in accordance with these rules we should have to infer, from a sufficient body of unprejudiced observation, that unprejudiced observation is a good guide to what lies beyond observation. But this claim is one that itself lies beyond observation, for it cannot be observed that unprejudiced observation is a good guide to what has not been, or cannot be, observed. Thus to infer from unprejudiced observation that such observation is a good guide to what lies beyond it we shall need to assume that such observation is a good guide to what lies beyond it. But this is the very assumption that we were hoping to *reach* in accordance with rules (a) and (b). Thus the attempt to reach this assumption by these rules gets absolutely nowhere, as it simply traps us in a circle. To put it another way, we cannot possibly inductively infer from observation the very assumption that is required by every inductive inference—for as it is required by every inductive inference it must be required by this inductive inference and so cannot (except in a circular fashion) be reached by inductive inference.

This result of Hume's completely devastates the inductivist's hope of demarcating empirical science from pseudoempirical superstition —for what it shows is that at the very heart of the inductive method lies an assumption that cannot be part of genuine empirical science. This assumption, often called the "principle of induction," turns out to be a preconceived idea, one that can receive empirical support only if it is first presupposed. But according to inductivism any such support is merely spurious, or pseudosupport, as it can be seen as support only in the light of the very idea that it is supposed to support. Thus the inductivist must, by his own rules, reject such a principle as a pseudoempirical superstition. But in that case empirical science, in so far as it is characterised by its use of inductive inference, must also be rejected as a pseudoempirical superstition and so cannot be demarcated from it.

Hume's result, which effectively shows that inductive inference cannot be part of empirical science, is not the only difficulty from which traditional inductivism suffers. Other problems abound. For example, modern psychological studies into the processes of perception make it quite clear that there is no such thing as the unprejudiced observation required by inductivism. Observation is always permeated with hypothetical, or theoretical, elements—for example, the perceptual phenomenon of size constancy requires the implicit assumption that objects do not get smaller as they move away from us.

For another example, the traditional requirement that inductive inference should be used only after we have collected a sufficient body of unprejudiced observations raises the crucial question of when our collected body of evidence is sufficient. It is clear that, in principle, we can go on observing for ever and that the observational evidence can never itself inform us of its own sufficiency. It follows that the inductivist can begin the process of learning from observation (by using inductive inference) only if he is willing to subscribe to the hypothesis that the observations already collected are sufficient for the purposes of inductive inference. But inductivism itself requires that such a hypothesis be rejected as an unscientific superstition, as it must be a mere anticipation or speculation because it could not possibly have been reached as a result of inductive inference. It follows once again that inductive learning from observation without hypotheses—that is, without preconceived ideas—is impossible, while learning from observation with such hypotheses is anathema to the inductivist.

Horns of a trilemma

In the light of the above considerations we find ourselves on the horns of a trilemma: either we continue to insist that what characterises empirical science is its use of the inductive method, in which case we must find some way round Hume's argument (and other difficulties); or we must conclude that empirical science is indeed just a pseudoempirical superstition; or we must find an alternative solution to the problem of demarcation.

Most contemporary philosophers of science refuse to countenance the possibility that the theories of empirical science are simply pseudoempirical superstitions. In this they are, I think, quite right. For let us assume that we equate empirical science with pseudoempirical superstition. We shall then have to conclude that the attempt to bring the benefits of Western medicine to other parts of the world is simply a matter of cultural imperialism as Western medical science is really no better than are the various traditional, usually superstitious, medical practices of others. Yet no one takes such a possibility seriously for a moment—least of all the inhabitants of the so called "underdeveloped world," who are, in the main, crying out for these benefits. Thus the idea, which might be taken to follow from Hume's result, that the theories of empirical science are simply pseudoempirical superstitions, on a par with primitive myths, witchcraft, or magic, is hardly acceptable to anyone.

Rejecting this horn of the trilemma thus leaves us with only two options: either we find some way round Hume's argument (and the other problems facing traditional inductivism) or else we find some alternative, non-inductivist, solution to the problem of demarcation. The overwhelming majority of contemporary philosophers of science adopt the first tack. This is not to say that they still harbour the hope that Bacon's theory of induction can be made to work. Quite the contrary: most acknowledge the impossibility of a Baconian inductive method by which a theoretical understanding and explanation of phenomena may be obtained directly from these phenomena by a process of inference. Nevertheless, they continue to hold that empirical science is, when compared with myths, superstitions, and so on, a particularly secure and reliable body of knowledge as it is somehow well supported by empirical evidence. They hope either that an inductive "logic of confirmation" can be made to work without resorting to any pseudoempirical assumption or principle (perhaps because it requires no more than the logical or mathematical assumptions of the calculus of probability—for example, Bayes's theorem) or that they can justify the use of induction pragmatically (as offering the best hope of achieving the aims of science).

Popper's non-inductivist solution

In opposition to all such attempts to salvage inductivism from the ravages of Hume's critique Sir Karl Popper[5-9] has suggested an elegant non-inductive solution to the problem of demarcation—one that enables us to explain, despite Hume's arguments, why the theories of

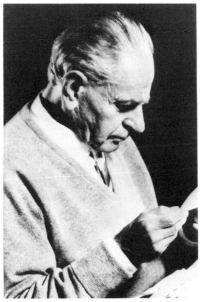

Karl Popper.

empirical science are to be preferred, from the point of view of truth, to those of witchcraft, scientology, and other pseudoempirical superstitions. According to Popper, what demarcates the theories of empirical science is not that they have been reached from observation by some special method of inference, or even that they are especially well supported by observation, but rather that they are open to observational and empirical criticism and refutation and that severe attempts have been made to discover their falsity by such means. Thus for Popper the distinguishing mark of empirical science is its insistence that only theories that are falsifiable—and hence testable—by empirical evidence be admitted; those that are admitted should then be subjected to the most severe and rigorous attempts at empirical elimination that we can devise.

Unlike traditional inductivism, Popper's solution to the problem of demarcation does not fall foul of Hume's criticism of inductive inference, for according to Popper empirical science has no need of inductive inference and so is not threatened by Hume's criticism of it.

To see this it is crucial to understand the very different role that empirical inquiry takes in Popper's view from that in the inductivist view. In traditional Baconian inductivism empirical inquiry is supposed to furnish us with the basis from which, by a process of inductive inference, the theories of empirical science are *reached*, while in contemporary inductivism empirical inquiry is supposed to furnish us with the basis on which the theories of empirical science are *supported*. In opposition to these views, Popper sees empirical inquiry as providing only the means by which the theories of empirical science are *tested*—where the aim of any test is to try to discover the falsity of our theories, not to support their claim to truth. As a theory cannot be tested unless it is already formulated there is no question here of trying to reach or infer theories from empirical evidence (for Popper our theories are our creations, our guesses, not the products of inference).

On the other hand, as the aim of any test is simply to discover whether our theories are false, and as every inference from the falsity of an empirical consequence of a theory to the falsity of the theory itself is a perfectly straightforward *deductive* inference, there is equally here no need for any inductive logic of confirmation or support. To put all this slightly differently, for Popper what present science tells us about the world has not been learnt from observation and experiment; rather, what we have learnt from observation and experiment is that much of what previous science tells us about the world is false. Thus we undoubtedly learn from our empirical inquiries, but what we have learnt is not what we know.

Now, recall that one way of formulating the problem of demarcation is as the question "How can we distinguish between genuine empirical support (or a genuine empirical method) and spurious, or pseudoempirical, support (or a pseudoempirical method)?" How does Popper's proposed solution help us with regard to this question? The answer is that it counsels us to stop looking for empirical support altogether and to direct our attention instead towards finding observable facts that may refute our theories. As we saw before, most superstitions—like the theories of witchcraft—can seem to be supported or confirmed by empirical or observational evidence. But the same can be said of false scientific theories, such as the phlogiston theory of combustion or the Ptolemaic theory of the heavens. The simple truth is that empirical support can be found for any theory, as long as we look for it. Thus the fact that a theory may agree with many observed facts should not be taken to indicate any virtue in the theory unless the facts have been obtained as a result of our attempts to refute the theory—that is, to show by empirical means that it is false.

In other words, spurious or pseudoempirical support results from the very desire to find empirical support; a genuine empirical method results only if we relinquish this desire and instead look for empirical refutations. Thus the fact that a theory that is open to refutation by empirical testing has survived our best efforts to discover its falsity allows us, quite rationally, to uphold its claim to truth (or at least its claim to being an approximation to truth); but the mere fact that a theory can be shown to agree with many observed facts says nothing whatsoever for its truth.

This point may become clearer if we consider a theory that is not open to empirical refutation at all—and which is thus, given Popper's proposed solution to the problem of demarcation, to be excluded from the realm of empirical science. Take, for example, the hypothesis that a certain house is haunted. This may be said to agree with many observed facts—for example, creaking doors, flickering lights, mysterious disappearances of food, intermittent interference on the telephone, and so on. If we uphold the view that a theory is worthy of serious consideration from the point of view of truth simply because it can be shown to agree with many observed facts then we shall have to conclude that this hypothesis is worthy of such consideration. Yet the contrary (and, I might add, equally untestable) hypothesis that the house is not haunted can also be shown to agree with many observed facts. But both cannot be true. In the absence of any empirical means of eliminating either of them as false the fact that both can be shown to agree with many observed facts says not a jot for the truth of either.

It is, I hope, clear from all this that Popper in fact agrees with Bacon that if we start from ideas (or hypotheses) there is a great danger that we will, like the witchdoctor, interpret evidence as confirmation of our ideas. But whereas Bacon taught that the solution to this problem lay in starting with observation and avoiding hypotheses Popper holds (in effect, following Hume) that we cannot avoid hypotheses if we hope to learn from observation. Thus the only way to avoid the danger is to stop valuing, and hence looking for, confirmation altogether and to insist instead on searching for empirical refutation. But once we insist on this search we will, quite naturally, want to focus our attention on those hypotheses that are open to such refutation and to exclude from empirical science those that are not.

From Popper's point of view, then, what renders the theories of empirical science worthy of serious consideration from the point of view of truth is not that we have good empirical grounds for believing their truth but rather that they are sensitive to eliminative empirical testing, that we have marshalled our best efforts in the attempt to show that they are not true, and that we have failed in this attempt. On the other hand, what renders the theories of witchcraft, scientology, and so on unworthy of serious consideration from the point of view of truth is not that there do not exist "good empirical grounds" for believing their truth (such "grounds" exist for every theory) but rather that they are immune to any attempt to refute them empirically or, if they are not so immune, are easily refuted as soon as the attempt is made.

Conclusion

Popper's solution to the problem of demarcation can, I suggest, explain the rationality of our preference for Western medicine over the superstitious medical practices of, for example, the witchdoctor. In so far as Western medical practice exploits scientific theories that, unlike the theories of witchcraft, are susceptible to empirical testing, have been severely tested, and have survived, and in so far as medicine has subjected its own independent techniques to severe empirical criticism (for example, in clinical trials) instead of merely looking for "positive instances," we have done everything that can be done to eliminate false theories and ineffective, or even harmful, techniques. This does not mean, of course, that we will thereby always get things right. Quite the contrary: the possibility of our making great new medical discoveries—and thus maintaining the superior intellectual status of medical science—will remain intact only as long as we are on the lookout for its shortcomings and are willing to modify and improve it in the light of consciously sought after failings. As Popper has aptly put it: "In politics and in medicine, he who promises too much is likely to be a quack."[10]

It is in this light that the recent report of the BMA on alternative medicine should be viewed. What is wrong with, say, faith healing is not that it does not have a "scientific basis" if this means that we cannot at present give any scientific explanation of its effectiveness. After all, it is perfectly possible that such practices are regularly effective in, say, curing cancer (just as the old wives' tale that milkmaids did not get smallpox turned out to be true). If this were the case then the fact that we cannot explain it within present medical science would not mean that faith healing is ineffective but rather that our present scientific knowledge is defective. But if the assertion that faith healing does not have any scientific basis means that the claims made on its behalf are incapable of being tested empirically, or have been subjected to such tests and have failed, this is quite a different matter. Of course, the defenders of faith healing may respond to any such negative findings by rejecting altogether the appropriateness of empirical tests for evaluating their claims; but in that case they are asking the rest of us to treat them as oracles, with an unimpeachable hotline to the truth.

If the history of medicine, and indeed of all science, teaches us anything it teaches us that there are no oracles. The history of our knowledge is replete with discarded and long forgotten theories. It follows that present medical science, however testable and well tested it is, is no oracle either. Popper's solution to the problem of demarcation can help us to understand why, despite this fact, we are right to accord greater intellectual status to the theories and practices of modern medical science than we do to those of witchcraft and the witchdoctor.

I gratefully acknowledge the financial support of the John Dewey Foundation at the Center for Dewey Studies, Southern Illinois University, Carbondale, Illinois, United States. Thanks are also due to David Miller, University of Warwick, for useful criticisms of an earlier version of this paper.

1 Heine H. Religion and philosophy in Germany. ([English translation 1882). Quoted in: Popper
   K. *The open society and its enemies*. Vol 2. London: Routledge and Kegan Paul, 1945:109.
2 Keynes JM. *The general theory of employment, interest, and money*. London: Macmillan, 1936:
   303-4.
3 Jarvie JC. Agassi J. The problems of the rationality of magic. In: Wilson B, ed. *Rationality*.
   Oxford: Blackwell, 1970:172-93.
4 Hume D. A treatise of human nature 1739. In: Selby-Biggs LA, ed. *Hume's treatise*. Oxford:
   Clarendon Press, 1888.
5 Popper KR. *The logic of scientific discovery*. London: Hutchinson, 1959.
6 Popper KR. *Conjectures and refutations*. London: Routledge and Kegan Paul, 1963.
7 Miller D, ed. *A pocket Popper*. London: Fontana, 1983.
8 Medawar P. Induction and intuition in scientific thought. In: *Pluto's republic*. Oxford: Oxford
   University Press, 1982.
9 Magee B. *Popper*. 2nd ed. London: Fontana, 1982.
10 Popper KR. *The open society and its enemies*. Vol 2. London: Routledge and Kegan Paul, 1945:
   334.

Formal logic and its applications in medicine

JOHN K SLANEY

Once upon a time the educated man (or, more rarely, woman) would have in his or her intellectual background, along with many Greek verbs and other curiosities, a smattering of logic. Logic, advertised as revealing the "laws of thought," was mainly a theory of syllogistic inference dating back as a system to the fourth century BC and in particular to Aristotle. It produced such useful and decorative specimens as:

> All Brazilians are footballers
> All footballers are bipeds
> Therefore all Brazilians are bipeds

—an instance of the valid syllogistic form known as "Barbara"[1] and enabled initiates to recognise and avoid the "undistributed middle" (a formal fallacy, not an unsightly condition brought on by hunching over textbooks). Its applicability to real life, however, was doubtful. Firstly, most of the really interesting reasoning going on was too advanced to be caught in the coarse mesh of a "tissue of syllogisms" being, for example, mathematical or analogical. Secondly, thought kept refusing to obey the "laws": only by jumping to conclusions, bending definitions, and the like can important progress be made in theorising, so that in describing anything like science logic labours along far behind life. Long before the intellectual explosion of the late nineteenth century that gave birth to modern medicine the study of formal logic had become an ingrown phenomenon. What kept it alive was not so much any theory that it offered of inference or rationality as the seductiveness of the patterns it made.

Divergence of medicine and logic

In the twentieth century logic and medicine have taken divergent paths. While medicine has emerged as a scientific discipline, sustained by unprecedented empirical success, merging at the edges not only with biology but with sciences from chemistry to psychology, and serving as a focus for technological innovation, logic has become an extremely abstract subject mainly serving the needs of pure mathematics and as distant from practical motivations as any academic concern. These different directions are historically explicable. Medicine responded to the possible when scientific theories of the origin and nature of diseases became well established and when modern drug technology and precision engineering emerged. Logic took its course because it was needed to help solve a crisis in the foundations of mathematics, and it stayed on to spawn new subjects of pure mathematical study.

This divergence was quite likely to have occurred anyway, given the nature of the subjects, under the pressure of the increasing depth of twentieth century inquiry with its consequent specialisation. It is wrong to bemoan the high degree of specialisation in current research. Although there is something disquieting about the thought of an extremely able mind engaged exclusively on a problem so minute that only the highly trained can see it, we should not forget that in a mature discipline only specialisation gets things done. What is genuinely pernicious is not narrowly delimited fields of inquiry but narrow vision blocking appreciation of anything outside the delimited field. I do not, of course, urge that medical practitioners all immediately take up mathematical logic or even suppose that a study of the mathematics of inference will make anyone a much better diagnostician—for that purpose empirical means tend to be more effective—but I do suggest that awareness of the abstract structure of theorising and decision making might contribute a degree of conceptual clarity, especially in those difficult circumstances in which the small steps of inference become important enough to be made explicit. I also want to indicate some ways in which recent developments in pure logic may be about to impinge on many other disciplines, medicine included.

Before this can be done it is necessary to describe formal logic. What follows is not intended to teach logic to anyone. There are many textbooks available,[1-3] and any interested reader should consult one of these for a proper introduction. Here I give only an overview, sketching in the conceptually important features in such a way that the later remarks make sense.

Valid or invalid?

Logic is concerned with arguments. An argument, like the one above about Brazilians and their feet, is not a dialogue but a record of a possible inference and consists of premises (two in the example, but any number, zero or more, in principle) and a conclusion, usually joined by "so" or "therefore." The premises and conclusion are statements and may be either true or false. An argument is valid if and only if there is no way that its premises could be true and its conclusion at the same time false. In a valid argument it is a matter of necessity that if the premises are true then so is the conclusion. Conversely, the argument is invalid if there is some possible situation that would make the premises true and the conclusions false. It is very important that there are valid arguments with false conclusions (and of course false premises):

> Pope John Paul II is a Scot
> All Scots support Rangers
> Therefore Pope John Paul II supports Rangers.

There are also invalid arguments whose premises and conclusions are all true:

> Pope John Paul II is a Christian
> All Catholics are Christians
> Therefore Pope John Paul II is a Catholic.

(Note that if the second premise were "All Christians are Catholics" the argument would be valid, though its premises would hardly be persuasive.) What there cannot be is a valid argument with true premises and a false conclusion.

Formal logic is the study not of individual arguments like those above but of abstractable features of language that enter systematically into questions of the validity or invalidity of argument forms. An argument form is the result of substituting variables for names, predicates, or even whole statements in an actual argument. It is valid if and only if every argument of that form is valid. Thus the above argument about Rangers is of the valid form:

> n is S
> All S are R
> Therefore n is R.

A certain amount of chopping and squeezing is needed to get natural arguments to fit such schematic forms. To judge the acceptability or unacceptability of the paraphrasing required, there is no alternative to native speakers' intuitions—a fact that, once noted, robs formal logic of the inexorability popularly associated with it.

The method used in formal logic is first to move away from everyday reasoning, setting up completely abstract mathematical systems codifying inference in simple artificial languages, and then to seek importance for the results by mapping back on to natural languages like English. The intended reading of a logical system will, of course, influence the choice of its language and rules but is not intrinsic to the system any more than possible physical applications of such mathematical constructions as group theory or geometry are parts of those properly mathematical theories.

Ifs and ands: a formal calculus

To illustrate the notion of a formal language for logic, and to be able to make certain observations later, I shall now present a simple logical system suitable for analysing the parts played in argument by two constructions: the conjunction "and" and the conditional "if . . . then. . . . " For these I shall use the notations "&" and "→," respectively. In the calculus given here we are not interested in the internal structure of statements not constructed with & and →, so we shall take an arbitrary set of such statements as atoms and write them as single letters, with superscripts if necessary: P, Q, R, P', Q', R', P''. . . . The connectives & and → may be applied repeatedly to these atoms to build up formulas of any complexity—for example, P & Q, R→R, (P & R)→(Q→ (P & P)), and so on. Here we have a language, a bit limited as languages usually go but sufficient to illustrate a few points.

We want to capture the valid forms of argument in our formal language. Because compounding under connectives is unlimited we should expect infinitely many valid forms, so listing them is not going to be helpful. What we do, therefore, is appeal to the notion of a formal derivation. To show that a given conclusion A follows from a set X of premises we produce a list $D_1, \ldots D_n$, A ending with A, each item in which is either one of the premises in the set X, or an immediate consequence derived from items earlier in the list by one of a small set of rules, or a subderivation in its own right. The rules defining "immediate consequence" and "sub derivation" will be specified below. First note how natural the idea of derivation is. An argument that may be complicated and unobvious is broken up by interpolating many small steps, each of which is simple and obvious and which only cumulatively provide the effect of complexity. Thus infinitely many argument forms may be reduced to a few very simple ones. This is the power of formal logic.

Ordinary proofs in mathematics are derivations in much the same sense given here. The argument whose premises are the axioms of Euclid's geometry and whose conclusion is Pythagoras's theorem, for example, is logically valid but far from obviously so; to make it convincing we interpose many simpler arguments whose validity is not in doubt. Ultimately, the derivation can be reconstructed in pure logic (though it needs a more elaborate system than the fragment presented here).

Rules of calculus

The precise rules governing & and → are fairly easily stated and justified. Firstly, any formula of the form A & B has the joint force of A and B. So:

Rule 1   A is an immediate consequence of A & B.

Rule 2   B is an immediate consequence of A & B.

Rule 3   A & B is an immediate consequence of A and B taken in either order.

These rules are given for all formulas A and B.

Secondly, to assert A→B (if A then B) is to claim a warrant for asserting B, given A. We can assert "If A then B" when we are in a position to infer B from A, perhaps together with other information we possess. So we may take it that the conditional A→B follows from the premises of an argument provided that if we took A as an extra premise we could derive B. This motivating thought gives rise to two more rules:

Rule 4   B is an immediate consequence of A→B and A in either order.

Rule 5   A→B is an immediate consequence of a subderivation with assumption A and conclusion B.

A subderivation is simply a derivation within a derivation, except that it must start with exactly one assumption (which may be any formula), whereas the main derivation starts with assumptions of all the premises. Items from any derivation may be used within any of its later subderivations, but items inside subderivations are not available from outside. Subderivations may be nested one inside the other to any finite depth.

Consider a couple of sample derivations to make all this clearer. First take the argument:

> If ice is placed in water it floats
> If ice is placed in water it melts
> Therefore if ice is placed in water it floats and melts.

This is boring but valid, as it can be regimented to fit the form P→Q, P→R, therefore P→(Q & R).

To prove this to be valid we derive its conclusion from its two premises thus:

(1)	P→Q	Premise
(2)	P→R	Premise
(3.1)	P	Assumption
(3.2)	Q	From 1 and 3.1 by rule 4
(3.3)	R	From 2, 3.1 by rule 4
(3.4)	Q & R	From 3.2 and 3.3 by rule 3
(4)	P→(Q & R)	From 3, by rule 5

Item three of the main derivation here is a subderivation with assumption P and conclusion Q & R. It is in turn composed of four items, 3.1 to 3.4, and is indented with a vertical line to make clear that it is a subderivation. Next consider the argument form (P & Q)→R, therefore P→(Q→R).

(1)	(P & Q)→R	Premise
(2.1)	P	Assumption
(2.2.1)	Q	Assumption
(2.2.2)	P & Q	From 2.1 and 2.2.1 by rule 3
(2.2.3)	R	From 1 and 2.2.2 by rule 4
(2.3)	Q→R	From 2.2 by rule 5
(3)	P→(Q→R)	From 2 by rule 5.

Here item 2.2 (composed of items 2.2.1 to 2.2.3) is a subderivation of item 2, which in turn is a subderivation of the main proof. The converse argument form P→(Q→R), therefore (P & Q)→R is also valid. The two together show the equivalence, for example, of: "If more blood is lost and no transfusion given the patient will die" to "If more blood is lost the patient will die without a transfusion."

This is not an appropriate place to dwell on the details of the fragment of formal logic just presented. Any interested reader will find other thorough expositions in a similar style.[23] The reason for giving it here is to provide an example, a target for pointing, to sustain the discussion that follows. Before passing to that discussion we should note the important concepts of interpretation, model, and theory.

Interpreting theories

To interpret a formal system is to give it a reading by assigning some values to the formulas (and in more advanced cases to other things, such as names and predicates). This will then produce an account of the meaning of the logical symbols (& and → in the example) in terms of their effects on the values of formulas and so on. Every interpretation picks out some set of formulas as being "true." If every formula in a set S is true for a given interpretation then that interpretation is said to be a model of S. A theory, in the sense provided by a formal logic, is a set of formulas in the appropriate language such that whenever any argument from $A_1 \ldots A_n$ to B is valid in the logic, and all of $A_1 \ldots A_n$ are in the theory, so is B. The items in a theory are called its theorems. A model of a theory is therefore an interpretation for which everything said by that theory is true.

For example, we can interpret our calculus of & and → in terms of the concept of "information." Suppose that there are some "pieces of information" and that we can pick out various sets of these as possible "states of information." It does not matter formally what these are: only the structure of the idea counts. One possible state of information —call it T (for True)—is supposed to be the information actually given by the real world. Now each atom (P, Q, and so on) is interpreted as conveying a piece of information. For a given interpretation in this sense each formula is either "warranted" or "not warranted" by each state of information as follows:

(1) An atom is warranted by state S if and only if its information is in S.

(2) A conjunction A & B is warranted by S if and only if both of A and B are warranted by S.

(3) A conditional A→B is warranted by S if and only if B is warranted by every state that includes S and warrants A.

A formula is true for an interpretation if and only if it is warranted by T according to that interpretation. An argument form is valid provided that its conclusion is true for every interpretation for which its premises are true. It can be shown that validity thus defined coincides with derivability according to the five rules given above in the sense that we get the same set of valid argument forms whether we define the logic as a system of derivations or as a theory of information. This fact is a completeness theorem for the system in question. This system differs slightly from the one more usually found in introductory texts, as will be noted below in section IV.

What has been set out in this section is, of course, a very small part of formal logic. It can be elaborated to take account of much more complex reasonings, including arguments of the kind given in section I and many others. Logical theory since 1900 has been partly a matter of formulating such elaborations and partly concerned with the investigation of concepts arising—the theory of sets, model theory, proof theory, parts of abstract algebra, recursion theory, and so on. Let us leave aside the technicalities of mathematical logic and return to considering the ways in which logic has to do with medicine.

Logic and life: the application of formal systems

Any science—physical, biomedical, or any other—has as its outcome theories. Theories may, as suggested in the last section, be considered as sets of statements closed under logic. Thus logic is the abstract theory of theories. A system of logic works on theories in two ways. Firstly, it issues permissions to argue in certain ways. It offers guarantees that certain forms of argument—the ones that it delivers as valid—will never introduce falsehood into any body of theory. Arguing in the permitted ways may bring hidden falsehoods to light but will not itself be the source of any error. Secondly, it prohibits certain sorts of theory. Specifically, it prohibits theories that do not contain all their own logical consequences. The significance of this fact will become apparent in the next section. In that it provides a characterisation of the concept of "theory," logic relates to medical science in just the same way as to other sciences, no more and no less closely.

A second way in which logic impinges on medicine is by imposing constraints on actual passages of argument. All rational activity is subject to rules; it is a virtue of the way in which it is governed by rules that it counts as rational. The rules of formal logic are culled from those of natural discourse and must be measured against such discourse to assess their adequacy. It is clear that valid and accurate reasoning is needed not only in research but also in the day to day practice of medicine—for instance, in diagnosis and in the decision making that goes with treatment. Much of this reasoning, where it is complex enough to need doing consciously, will require far more elaborate parts of language than are covered by the example of & and → calculus given above. It will be partly mathematical, particularly probabilistic, for instance. But its basic structure will still be logical, and there is no reason why reflective awareness of the qualitative logical structure of inference should not add some clarity to the thought processes required. At the very least, fluency with formal languages often confers a facility in grasping and manipulating intricate or convoluted statements or reasonings, keeping track of several layers of hypothesis, and so on.

Counterexample

A system of formal logic is a catalogue of valid forms of inference, but it is not going to be used as a straightforward diagnostic tool like a chart or handbook. Appeals to logic occur in more complicated dialectical contexts. Suppose, for example, someone makes a claim C, of which you are unconvinced. You may well reply by asking why C is thought to be true. Its proponent might then produce an argument with C as its conclusion. At this point you have several rational options. One option is to challenge the validity of the argument, perhaps backing up your challenge with a counterexample—that is, another argument of the same form but with true premises and a manifestly false conclusion. For example, if the proffered argument were:

> If there is an Act of God on Saturday United stand a chance
>   of winning
> There will be no Acts of God this week
> Therefore United don't stand a chance

a suitable counterexample might be the parallel argument:

> If Edinburgh is part of Glasgow it is in Scotland   (true)

Edinburgh is not part of Glasgow	(true)
Therefore Edinburgh is not in Scotland.	(false)

If the argument were:

No car is dangerous unless badly driven
Jimmy drives a Porsche very badly
Therefore Jimmy's car is dangerous

we could counter that you might as well argue:

No car is legal unless it has brakes	(true)
Jimmy drives a wreck with brakes	(suppose true)
Therefore Jimmy's car is legal.	(false, as it has bald tyres and no lights)

A counterexample, however, may not end the debate, as there is room for disagreement about whether the two arguments are really of the same form, whether the first is also of some other, valid, form, and so on.

One direction that the discussion could then take would be an appeal by the proponent of C to formal logic. An argument form might be found that is provable in the formal system and whose conclusion fits the form of C. This is what Euclid did in geometry with problematic propositions like Pythagoras's theorem, as already noted. The debate, however, might still not end, for you have the options of criticising the formalisation—the mapping between natural and formal language—and of course of denying or questioning one or more premises of the formalised argument. You might even question the correctness of the formal system itself, as we shall see. The debate over support for C can go on for a long time, getting more and more convoluted. Appeals to logic may sometimes settle the matter; sometimes they bear on it less directly by exposing hidden assumptions, contentious definitions, and the like, advancing understanding of what is at stake. Much of philosophy, natural theology, and (more frivolously) the activities of the Flat Earth Society show the lengths to which this kind of rational investigation may go. Lakatos provides an illuminating and profound discussion, in delightful style, of some of the intricacies arising particularly in mathematical reasoning.[4]

Philosophy of medicine

Questions demanding definitions can easily lead to investigations into the conceptual foundations of medicine. Think of simple questions such as "Is the common cold one disease with many causes or many diseases with similar symptoms?" This may seem to be fairly trivial, but it quickly leads to harder issues such as: How may diseases be individuated? Have biological discoveries taught us more about diseases or have they given us a new concept of "disease"? Is the concept of a disease useful at all? As there is in any case no treatment (apart from lessening the symptoms) what purposes, if any, are served by the possible finer distinctions?

In approaching questions of this sort we are no longer studying medicine but studying the philosophy of medicine. Medical explanations are another source of philosophical tangles. Consider the old joke about the patient with the arthritic hip:

DOCTOR: How old are you?

PATIENT: 82.

DOCTOR: Well then, it's probably due to old age.

PATIENT: Can't be. The other hip's just as old, and there's nothing wrong with that.

The joke rests on a misunderstanding of the way in which the explanation is to be taken. What does it show about the concept of explanation in medicine? How does such explanation compare with explanation in natural science? In the social sciences? In everyday life? Answers to questions like these cannot simply be read off a formal logical calculus, but logical reasoning will certainly be required if they are pursued seriously.

The future: logic in computation

One way in which logic is going to be important to medicine is through the impact of computer technology. Because the factual basis of medicine is so immense and detailed, and because the day to day diagnostic and other problems it poses are set up in terms of these complex empirical facts, observed symptoms, case histories, known effects of treatments, and so on, medicine is a natural home for what are now becoming known as knowledge based expert systems. The science fiction dream of a robot doctor, a specialist in everything, is closer to reality than was thought possible even a few years ago. Not, perhaps, the smartly dressed tin man with the perfect bedside manner but the micro in the corner of the surgery with access to a database equal in information content to the accumulated knowledge of many specialists; this is just next year's handy gadget. Next year? Well, perhaps the year after; certainly within a decade. The necessary hardware—cheap, fast microprocessors, compact discs, and so on—is either in the shops now or just about to be. Many aspects of the software still need much work, but progress is reported almost constantly. Clearly, some knowledge based systems will soon be common, and their scope and their automatic reasoning ability will increase manyfold over the next few years.

Artificial intelligence

The theory of computation is in part an offshoot of mathematical logic. It has recently been joined by another offshoot: the new science of artificial intelligence. "Expert" systems addressing large bases of data need to be artificially intelligent to some degree. In particular, to arrive at answers to unforeseen questions they have to make deductions using the data as premises. For this purpose they have to use some sort of logic. An expert system must, therefore, be in part an inference system.

Thus formal logic is about to re-enter the practical sphere in a very important way through developments in artificial intelligence. In the remainder of this paper I want to outline just one aspect of the new development of logic, showing how certain abstruse reflections coming from philosophical logic could turn out to be pertinent to these very practical matters. Such relevance cannot readily be predicted and is one of the urgent reasons why basic research needs to be fostered without much reference to short term profits or visible products.

Recall that systems of logic like that set out on pp 20-23 are intrinsically simply abstract algebras. They gain their importance from analogies between their formal rules and reasoning processes in real life. There are at least two reasons why this leaves it rather indeterminate whether a given formal system is a correct account of logic. Firstly, there are just not enough facts about natural reason to settle all the questions. Real life reasoning is not that precise. Secondly, logic is a theory not about how people do reason but about how they ought to reason. Thus adopting a system of formal logic as a template for arguing, theorising, and the like will tend to influence the rules actually in force governing rationality.

To illustrate the indeterminacy of logic consider the argument:

If if grass is green then snow is white then grass is green
Therefore grass is green.

If you have any firm intuitive sense of whether this is valid or not then you are on your own. The corresponding argument form $(P{\rightarrow}Q){\rightarrow}P$, therefore P is invalid in the system set out in section II but valid according to the account of $\rightarrow$ more usually offered by logicians. How can the issue be decided? Certainly not by appealing to one off intuitions. Formal logical investigations will show that it makes a large systematic difference which way we decide, and philosophically based preferences may then sway us one way or the other. The mathematical and philosophical publications on this point are many and mostly rather abstruse, though Van Dalen gives a good account of the issues.[5] Argument forms like the one above get labelled valid or invalid on the basis of some larger theory, not on their individual merits; different choices of theory may well label them differently.

Deviant logic

Led by reflections like these or by convictions that the usual logical theories were in error, logicians of adventurous dispositions have developed many rival formal systems and offered them as being more or less adequate reconstructions of natural reasoning. Over the past hundred years or so there has been a steady growth both in the number of well investigated alternative systems made available and in the realisation of how wide the choice of logics is. Research in non-standard logic, however, has always been a minority interest, tending to be regarded by mathematicians as philosophical dabbling and by philosophers as mathematics gone awry. "Deviant" logic has never been a quick road to academic tenure. Recently, however, the situation has begun to change since the arrival of computer scientists who have practical problems to solve, no axes to grind, and no particular resistance to the idea that logical theorems might be open to question. At least two groups of "deviant" logicians are becoming recognised as having much to offer to the new science of automated reasoning. They are the advocates of "fuzzy logic" and of "relevant logic."

The guiding notion of fuzzy logic is that truth and falsehood, rather than being all or nothing, are matters of degree. In models for this kind of logic there is a continuum of values between absolute truth and absolute falsehood, so that on interpretation statements can lie vaguely in a middle range. Associated with fuzzy logic are fuzzy theories. Fuzzy set theory is particularly important and gives rise to theories of fuzzy functions, fuzzy numbers, and so on.[67]

Quite apart from the advantages of sensitivity to the vagueness typical of most of natural language, fuzzy values are useful in representing information that is either imprecise or true or false to a degree, or both, but that does not involve probabilities. Descriptions of medical symptoms are often of this kind: degrees of severity, extensiveness, persistence, and so on, are very important and are more readily mapped formally on to fuzzy values than on to probabilities. There is a lively debate among users of the theory of information retrieval systems over the merits of a basis of fuzzy logic for evaluating descriptions of items in a database.[6] Although the issue is by no means settled and is unlikely to be settled quickly, claims made for the increased accuracy and suitability of responses in fuzzy based systems at least need to be met. With or without a fuzzy logic probability theory is necessary for any formal reconstruction of diagnostic logic. The intricacies of combining probabilities with fuzzy reasoning are generating further, often difficult, research.

Relevant logic is harder to characterise briefly. It differs from orthodox logic in not allowing as valid those arguments whose premises are not related in subject matter to their conclusions.[58] An example is P, therefore Q→Q, proved as follows:

(1)	P		Premise
(2.1)		$\lfloor$Q	Assumption for subproof
(3)	Q→Q		From 2, by rule 5.

Proofs like this are blocked in relevant logic by the requirement that premises be used before anything counts as a derivation from them. Specifying what is a "use" turns out to be a delicate matter. The formal development of relevant logics is also complicated, their model theory especially presenting difficulties.

That relevant logic is a stable and workable system that is weaker than orthodox logic—that is, allowing fewer inferences—turns out quite unexpectedly to be useful. As the logic is weaker than usual it prohibits fewer kinds of theory than usual and has more models than usual. At the same time relevant logic is strong enough to allow the reconstruction of most—arguably all—of the proofs that anyone actually needs. In constructing automated reasoning systems it is advantageous to use a logic no stronger than necessary, because automatic reasoning is not so much a matter of driving derivations forward along valid lines as of avoiding attempts to reach conclusions by means that are not going to work. The automated reasoner looks at the desired conclusion and asks how such a thing could have been derived. There are usually many possible answers to try out, and the trick is to reject false trails as efficiently as possible in order to leave the correct one.

Discovering that a possible route leads nowhere is often a very complex and difficult matter. One way to make it simple is to use an interpretation of the logic in which counterexample to the proposed derivation is exposed. And the more models—especially "small" ones—that the logic has the more chance there is for this strategy to succeed. Some of the extra models are wildly unintended but show easily that theories have intended properties. For example, relevant arithmetic has an interpretation in which $0=2$. This is absurd, of course, but none the less suitable for showing that we cannot relevantly prove $0=1$ (something surprisingly difficult for orthodox arithmetic). As automated reasoning is so much a matter of avoiding the unprovable, rather than advancing directly to proofs, systems in which disproofs are easy to determine could well be more efficient than their orthodox counterparts. Again, the practical investigations and the debate over their use are at an early stage, but at least some results seem to be non-trivial.[9]

Unorthodox benefits

I do not wish to give the impression that research in unorthodox logic is the only or even the main source of what is valuable in artificial intelligence. The two examples just given are intended to show how research programmes that have confused and impractical beginnings may bear unexpected fruit. Both relevant and fuzzy logic grew out of philosophical concerns of at best debatable intrinsic worth and have been pursued for years by small groups well outside the mainstream of research in logic. Yet both are now set to deliver insights beneficial to information technology and thus to its applications, including those in medicine. Both illustrate the view of logic that I have tried to present throughout this essay. Formal logic is not a technique for making diagnosis easier, though it does bear obliquely on that problem. It is an abstract and beautiful study of how the attempt to describe reality is self coherent. Practical applications arise indirectly, sometimes from its most unlikely facets.

When I was first asked to write an article outlining my subject for a medical audience I confess to having found the prospect daunting, standing as I do a little in awe of the sheer volume of knowledge characteristic of medicine in contrast with the pure speculation more often found in logical research. Having arrived at this end of the business, I hope to have caused people to have some new and perhaps unfamiliar thoughts. And of course if anyone reading this is moved to develop an interest in logic or its kindred disciplines the task was worth doing.

1 Kneale W, Kneale M. *The development of logic*. Oxford: Oxford University Press, 1962:232.
2 Fitch FB. *Symbolic logic; an introduction*. New York: Ronald Press, 1952.
3 Kalish D, Montague R. *Logic: techniques of formal reasoning*. New York: Harcourt, Brace and World, 1964.
4 Lakatos I. *Proofs and refutations*. Cambridge: Cambridge University Press, 1976.
5 Gabbay D, Guenther F. *Handbook of philosophical logic*. Vol III. Dordrecht: Reidel, 1985.
6 Orlowska E, Wierzchon S. Mechanical reasoning in fuzzy logics. *Logique et Analyse* 1985;**110**: 193-207.
7 Schmucker KJ. *Fuzzy sets, natural language computations and risk analysis*. Maryland: Computer Science Press, 1984.
8 Anderson AR, Belnap ND. *Entailment: the logic of relevance and necessity*. Vol I. Princeton: Princeton University Press, 1975.
9 Thistlewaite PB, Meyer RK, McRobbie MA. Advanced theorem-proving techniques for relevant logics. *Logique et Analyse* 1985;**110**:233-56.

Diagnostic logic

FERGUS J MACARTNEY

The history of diagnostic logic must be as old as that of medicine itself; the motivation to improve it has probably never been stronger than it was in the mind of the caveman patient as he felt the rasp of the trepan drilling a hole in his skull. Was the hole there to let the disease out or the cure in? Doctors have always been fascinated by diagnosis and the means by which it can be reached, but until recently the purpose of studying diagnostic logic has simply been to improve thought processes. Today this remains the primary objective, but a second motive becomes ever more important—namely, that of computer modelling of the diagnostic process.

Firstly, however, we have to consider how we may measure the usefulness of a method of diagnosis. That it should be sufficiently accurate goes almost without saying, but I would like to suggest that brevity (or, to be more specific, parsimony) is the second most important criterion by which a diagnostic process should be judged.

There is here a clear analogy with mathematical proofs. Two methods may be used to prove the same theorem, but that which always brings joy to the heart of the mathematician is the shorter and neater. This can, of course, be overdone. The great Johann Karl Friedrich Gauss, for example, when challenged as to how he had arrived at the conclusion of one of his exquisitely brief theorems, would reply loftily, "When a beautiful cathedral is built, who wants to see the scaffolding?" His proofs were indeed so short that they were often disbelieved. This did wonders for the curricula vitae of the next generation of lesser mathematicians, who published numerous lengthier proofs of what Gauss had already shown.

33

Is diagnosis necessary?

If we pursue the virtue of parsimony sufficiently ruthlessly we reach the interesting conclusion that under certain circumstances diagnosis is a pointless or meaningless diversion in the therapeutic process, which is, after all, the one that interests the patient. As a first example, take the question of whether a patient who has acute pain in the abdomen has appendicitis or Meckel's diverticulitis. Provided that the affected structure is in its usual position the precise diagnosis has no effect whatever on the management of the patient. It is the decision to perform a laparotomy through an incision in the right iliac fossa that matters.

As a second example, take the man aged 45 who has a blood pressure of 130/87 mm Hg. The question "Does this patient have hypertension?" is pointless, as it assumes that patients either have or do not have hypertension, whereas all that they have is different degrees of increased blood pressure. The key questions are not diagnostic but prognostic—namely, is this patient at increased risk of death, stroke, or other complications, and if so will the benefits of antihypertensive treatment or the search for a directly treatable cause, or both, outweigh the costs?

Finally, consider the value of psychiatric diagnosis, a subject on which whole books have been written.[1] I recall as an undergraduate being alternately fascinated and astonished by the teaching of William Sargent. Into his outpatient department would come a man enshrouded by an almost palpable aura of gloom; we would be told rather unnecessarily that he was depressed. Next through the door would come a woman who looked as if she had just won a parliamentary election, even though she was anxious about the possibility of there being a recount.

"Ah, another classical example of depression," would declare the master. It took a brave student indeed to ask how two such different people could possibly be suffering from the same disease.

"Simple, the lady has atypical depression," we would be told. I have to confess that my nerve failed me at this point, and I dared ask no more. Ultimately, the truth dawned. Patients who had classical endogenous depression responded to drugs that were self evidently antidepressant. If patients who had other symptoms responded to antidepressant drugs then they must be depressed. Simple, really. However illogical the argument, Sargent was trying to maintain that what mattered was to recognise which patients would respond to different forms of treatment, rather than to argue over the truth of the diagnosis with which their problem was labelled.

Thus though I would agree with Wulff that "the clinician today must recognise that the present disease taxonomy is arbitrary, imperfect and everchanging,"[2] I think that it is necessary to qualify the second half of his sentence, which reads: "at the same time he must realise that we cannot do without it." This may be true in general, but it certainly is not true in particular. Furthermore, this paradox arises precisely from the arguments that Wulff, Scadding, and Campbell have put forward so well.[2-4] Disease spotting is in some respects like bird spotting, but while birds can exist in isolation diseases cannot. To be sure, a tubercle bacillus can be isolated from a patient who is sick with tuberculosis, and a ventricular septal defect is a ventricular septal defect be it inside or outside the body, but both of these are diagnosed in the first instance because of their manifestations in sick patients. We may look on our therapeutic objective as killing the tubercle bacillus or closing the ventricular septal defect, but this has no value unless we make the sick patient better. Furthermore, this disease centred approach breaks down with something like rheumatoid arthritis, as it is at present not possible to separate the disease from the patient. Our only therapeutic objective is to make the sick patient better, so this may or may not include "naming" the disease.

In a passage of great profundity, Campbell points out the following: "A disease is first recognised syndromally—a constellation of clinical features. The disease has a cause (infective, nutritional, genetic, immunological, etc); this cause produces characteristic structural changes, which in turn produce the clinical manifestations. The elucidation of the causative, structural and functional changes may not come in any particular historical order, but the paradigm has two characteristics: first, it is expected or at least hoped the relations will be specific (unique cause, unique structural and functional changes belonging to one syndrome); second, as knowledge progresses, the defining process is 'pushed to the left' in the sequence given above. In other words, a disease will not be allowed to remain in syndromal terms if it can be explained or defined in functional terms; a functional syndrome will not be left in these terms if it can be characterised structurally, and 'cause' takes priority overall."[4]

It follows that, though precise diagnosis may be unnecessary for parsimonious treatment of the patient (as I have shown), it probably remains essential for the "pushing to the left" process just described.

Furthermore, though it might be imagined that precise diagnosis could be most easily dispensed with at the messy syndromal stage, which is characterised by endless futile discussion about what constitutes the syndrome (for example, depression), diagnosis can in fact be conveniently forgotten even after considerable pushing to the left, as at the functional (for example, hypertension) or even the structural stage (for example, appendicitis versus Meckel's diverticulitis).

The diagnostic process

From this point on we shall assume that diagnosis is a desirable end. Though many doctors love to imagine that diagnosis is some mystical process beyond logical analysis (this makes of them an elite priesthood), the fact is that hunch and intuition are unteachable, whereas logic can be taught. Furthermore, computers are logical but totally unimaginative.

The blunderbuss approach

The blunderbuss approach is the traditional method taught to medical students. They take a detailed history, examine the patient from top to toe, and then order every test that could conceivably have some bearing on the problem. Not until all the information is to hand do they try and work out what is the matter with the patient. This is done by fitting the pattern of abnormalities found either to textbook descriptions of diseases or to their own database of diseases in patients whom they have previously seen.

The nearest automated approach to the blunderbuss method is that of database comparisons.[5] An interactive search is made of a large database of information on patients, looking for those who match the particular patient under consideration. Usually a match is first sought on a limited list of features, with the result that a rather large and inhomogeneous subset of matching patients is obtained. The number of features to be matched is then increased, and the subset usually becomes smaller. When a matching subset is obtained in which the disease diagnosed in all patients is the same the new patient is assumed to have the same disease and can then be added to the database.

This method requires the accumulation of a large database free from errors, which is very expensive, yet there is no real concept within it of a list of possible diagnoses, each having a different probability of being true. Probably the most suitable application is in the diagnosis of rare syndromes,[6] where there is a real problem of human memory and collation of small snippets of information from diverse sources. Cases can be added from reports in journals as well as from the experience of collaborating centres, thus pooling information that could never effectively be accommodated in the memory of a single clinician.

This clinical approach is woefully unimaginative, cumbersome, and extravagant (as opposed to parsimonious). When applied to laboratory tests it wastes money, not only because many of the tests originally ordered are unnecessary but also because the more tests that are ordered the more likely it is that, by chance, one or more will turn out to be "abnormal" and start a wild goose chase of further tests to investigate the chance abnormality.

If this method is so bad why does it continue to be taught? Why are students not encouraged to use searchlights rather than buckets, to borrow a phrase from Popper? Part of the reason is that a searchlight cannot be used effectively without a fairly thorough knowledge of the territory to be searched. Students need to familiarise themselves with the normal as well as the abnormal. It is good practice for them to examine the whole patient every time. A thorough history taking and physical examination is also a cheap screening test for unsuspected disease not associated with the particular problem that has brought the patient to the doctor.

A further reason for the blunderbuss method continuing to be taught is that should an unfortunate doctor ever appear before a court he is far more likely to be criticised for sins of omission than sins of commission. Until lawyers learn the virtue of parsimony and understand that medical decisions are made on the basis of uncertainty, not matters "beyond reasonable doubt," medical education will continue to be blighted accordingly.

Algorithmic diagnosis

Algorithmic diagnosis will not be described in detail, as the *BMJ* has recently published series of clinical algorithms. These consist of a series of questions linked by lines labelled with the answers, which lead either to the next question, or, less often, to the diagnosis.[7] There is one entry point to the algorithm, and if the questions are followed through a diagnosis will be reached. The same diagnosis may be reached by several different routes.

The idea of clinical algorithms comes, ironically, from a rather unfashionable method of computer programming known as flow chart construction. Flow charts were devised to mimic the Boolean logic that is "built in" to digital computers and consists in essence of manipulating the logical operators *and*, *or*, and *not* in *if* statements (for example, *if* it is snowing *and* the fountains are turned off in Trafalgar Square *then* it is New Year's Eve).

Algorithmic approaches to diagnosis are exemplified by programs for evaluating acid-base disorders[8] and comatose patients.[9] If an algorithm is sufficiently simple there is no point in computerising it; it is quicker and simpler to follow a printed version of the original algorithm.

As will be discussed, algorithms are often rather gross oversimplifications of the diagnostic process. This has led to a broadening out of the concept into production rule systems by experts in artificial intelligence.[10 11] The comparison of databases and statistical systems requires a database of patients that is expensive and time consuming to obtain. By contrast, production rule systems require a database of knowledge consisting of production rules that are Boolean statements of the kind already described. The attraction of this approach to systems analysts is immediately obvious. Instead of spending years accumulating boring data on patients they can spend an afternoon with medical experts, picking their brains until they have translated their expertise into a series of production rules. The result has been diagnostic programs such as those for glaucoma (Casnet/glaucoma)[12] and neurological localisation in unconscious patients.[13]

The great advantage of clinical algorithms is their predictability. If the same set of information is fed into them the same answer will always emerge. The problem is that real life is seldom that simple. For this reason I believe that algorithms are best devised by experts for the use of non-experts. One of the most difficult judgments that an expert has to make is how seriously to take the information and conclusions given by an unfamiliar non-expert who consults her about a patient. If the non-expert has used an algorithm with which the expert is familiar, and that algorithm is based on observations that are reproducible even in the hands of non-experts, then the expert is much better to evaluate the information. She may know, for example, that the diagnosis given by the algorithm is not certain, but at least she should be able to judge how uncertain it is.

The Boolean example of New Year's Eve given above shows one of the most serious difficulties of the production rule approach. It is not quite certain that it is New Year's Eve just because it is snowing and the fountains are turned off. Thus some measure of uncertainty is required that is propagated from one rule to another. Attempts to do this so far[12 14] seem to be naive to statisticians,[15] who after all are old hands at quantifying uncertainty. Other serious problems with this approach are the difficulties of encompassing medical knowledge in production rules[13] and of being sure that these production rules are being applied in appropriate circumstances.[14]

The hypotheticodeductive model

The two models just discussed were almost diametrically opposite, but both were unsatisfactory. The key elements in the hypotheticodeductive model are the generation and testing of hypotheses, which together form a well recognised pattern of adult thinking.[16] The importance of this model in diagnosis was probably first put forward by Campbell.[17 18] It is attractive precisely because it allows for hunch and intuition in the diagnostic process, as these may be the source of hypotheses generated. None of the other models discussed here do this. Equally, this is the only model that cannot be programmed into a computer without sacrificing one of its most important characteristics. Campbell[4] asserts emphatically that his understanding of diagnosis springs from a Popperian view of scientific discovery,[19] but it is important to realise that there are some aspects in which the hypotheticodeductive model departs substantially from the Popperian approach. Although there is almost complete agreement on the importance of the generation of hypotheses and the sources of hypotheses, the Popperian view of how hypotheses should be tested is far too narrow for diagnostic purposes. These two opposing points will now be expanded.

The classical inductive view of science has no room for imagination but regards the foundation of scientific knowledge as consisting of particular observations (including experiments) from which general laws of the universe can be induced. The Popperian view is attractive in that it does not accept that scientists are passive observers but rather sees them as actively generating hypotheses to be tested, very often using their imaginations to do so. The generation of hypotheses is clearly identifiable in the behavioural analyses of clinicians at work[20][21] and begins remarkably early, often as soon as the clinician is aware of the complaint, age, and sex of the patient. To give a well known example, the clinician seeing a fat fertile woman aged 40 immediately hypothesises that she has gall stones.

Once this rather romantic Popperian view of science is grasped it becomes easier to understand the subtlety of a celebrated quotation by Medawar: "In commencement addresses and other uplifting declarations, clinicians who discourse on the 'spirit of medicine' will always point out that, while there is a large and profoundly important scientific element in the practice of medicine, there is also an indefinable artistry, an imaginative insight, and medicine (they will tell us) is born of a marriage between the two. But then (it seems to me) the speaker spoils everything by getting the bride and groom confused. It is the unbiased observation, the apparatus, the ritual of fact finding and the inductive mumbojumbo that the clinician thinks of as 'scientific', and the other element, intuitive and logically unscripted, which he thinks of as a creative art."[22]

Testing hypotheses forms an important part of both the classical inductive and the Popperian deductive approaches to the foundations of scientific knowledge. While the inductive approach regards testing hypotheses as including both verification and falsification of the hypothesis, however, Popper insists that only falsification increases knowledge.[19] The reason for this is that if verification is held to validate a hypothesis the assumption is that whatever experiment is being used to verify the hypothesis it will always give the same result, however often it is repeated. This is a matter of faith in the orderliness of creation, not of objectively demonstrable fact. Either you accept that it is a matter of faith or you conclude that the only acceptable way of testing a hypothesis is to prove it to be false. This is not as nihilistic as it first sounds, because scientific knowledge is advanced if an alternative hypothesis is put forward that contains more information and yet explains all the observations made so far. This new hypothesis is better because it contains more information, but it is not "the truth" because it survives only until it too is disproved.

It is clear from the observational studies already quoted that in clinical diagnosis the evaluation of hypotheses consists of both verification and falsification.[21] Indeed, were clinicians to insist on falsifying every hypothesised diagnosis save one an enormous amount of time would be wasted, and the principle of parsimony already alluded to would be violated. Are clinicians therefore anti-Popperian? Not necessarily. It is just that when we seek to diagnose the problem in a patient we are not in the business of establishing the foundations of scientific knowledge. To do that we require certainty (that a hypothesis is false, according to Popper). From a practical point of view, to diagnose the problem we do not have to be certain that the diagnosis is correct. All we need to know is that if we manage the patient on the assumption that this diagnosis is correct the patient will do better than if any other diagnosis is assumed. This point is foundational. Failure to understand it lies behind much muddled thinking on diagnosis.

We shall return in due course to the question of how we may be sure that a diagnosis is sufficiently accurate, but to avoid confusion it should be emphasised that what has just been written refers to the optimal management of an individual patient. Other considerations enter once we have other objectives, such as generalisations based on populations that have a particular disease. It has already been shown that diagnostic differentiation between appendicitis and Meckel's diverticulitis is not necessary for appropriate management of the patient with acute abdomen. To make generalisations about Meckel's diverticulitis, however, it is important that the diagnosis should be established as stringently as possible. Indeed, it can be argued that the less well defined a disease is the more important it is to make an accurate diagnosis.[1] The recognition by psychiatrists of the unreliability of psychiatric diagnosis led some to argue that psychiatric diagnosis should be abandoned.[23] But if this is done all hope for advancing knowledge of psychiatric illness disappears, as there is no means by which the foundation of diagnosis can be pushed to the left—that is, from the syndromic to the functional, anatomical, and causal. What is required is more reliable methods of diagnosis, not abandonment of the concept.

Much has been made so far of the place of imagination in generating hypotheses. In reality, most hypotheses arise from more prosaic sources, which have been well described by Cutler.[24] These include recognising patterns of varying degrees of complexity. There are trilogies (weight loss, exophthalmos, and tachycardia suggest thyrotoxicosis), tetralogies (squatting, hypoxic spells, cyanosis, and right ventricular hypertrophy suggest Fallot's tetralogy), and more complicated combinations of signs. These are rather amenable to computer based diagnosis, in contrast to what might be termed monologies, where the problem is diagnosed as the patient walks into the room. The facial appearances of patients who have Down's syndrome and idiopathic hypercalcaemia syndrome are so characteristic to an experienced clinician that it is doubtful whether either should be referred to as a syndrome. Certainly the term Down's syndrome should be dropped once the chromosomes have been examined, for this allows anatomical diagnosis.

There seems to be good evidence that the limited short term memory of the clinician means that the number of hypotheses entertained at any one time is restricted to four $\pm$ one.[25] Thus rejection of hypotheses is helpful not only in its own right but as a means of conserving short term memory. Once the hypothesis has been rejected it may be forgotten.

The hypotheticodeductive model forms the basis of what are termed cognitive programs.[26] The complexity of the approach is well illustrated by Pauker et al.[27] The clearest analogue to recognising sets (for example, tetralogies) is probably in the set covering model,[28] which is also capable of handling the difficult problem of multiple simultaneous disorders. The most ambitious of these programs is probably Internist,[29] which has developed into Caduceus[30] and covers 500 general medical diseases and over 3500 "manifestations."

Although there is much that is attractive in the hypotheticodeductive model, it has important drawbacks. Firstly, there is no real concept of the cost of evaluating hypotheses. In fact, much time and money is wasted on doing laboratory tests to rule out diagnoses that are extremely unlikely anyway or to confirm diagnoses that are already as certain as they need to be. This probably explains why the model fits history taking much more effectively than physical examination[26] or laboratory investigation. Questions cost nothing.

Secondly, there is no adequate explanation of the value of new information; as we shall see, this is much more subtle a matter than simply confirming or refuting hypotheses.

Thirdly, from the point of view of computer modelling (and this applies to expert systems in general) the question has to be asked whether the objective should be to mimic clinicians or to use computers to do the things that clinicians cannot do in their heads (such as multivariate analysis). I understand the motivation of those working with computers who wish to mimic the brain, but I as a doctor want a system that will do better than the best clinician. A machine that simply does what a clinician (even a superb clinician) does is simply not a very attractive proposition.

Finally, the argument that "this is what good clinicians do; therefore it is the best model available" may not be sound. Perhaps what good clinicians do reflects how they were trained in diagnosis and they would do better if trained differently.

Bayesian probability revision

Diagnostic logic owes more than most doctors probably imagine to the work of an eighteenth century English clergyman, Thomas Bayes. When not on his pastoral duties, Bayes indulged in his hobby, mathematics; would that more clinicians were as versatile. It is impossible to discuss Bayes's theorem without introducing mathematics, but to reduce the shock I shall first give an example of diagnostic logic as it applies to my own subject, paediatric cardiology, and then show that the approach is analogous to successive applications of Bayes's theorem. This approach to diagnostic logic was learnt by myself and many others at the feet of that gifted teacher of adult cardiology, David Mendel, long before I (and probably he) knew anything about Bayes or his theorem. Similarly, I have taught this method to a generation of housemen and registrars without reference to Bayes except where some aptitude to mathematics is evident.

League table diagnosis

Phase 1—A child is referred to me as an outpatient. Into my mind comes a league table of ranked probabilities, starting with the highest. Top of the league is innocent systolic murmur, followed in order by venous hum, bicuspid aortic valve, ventricular septal defect, atrial septal defect, and patent ductus arteriosus. The ranking comes from their incidence in the population referred to me. Below patent ductus is an extremely long list, the details of which do not matter.

Phase 2—The mother brings the child in, and I observe that the child is a baby of 3 months old. This immediately knocks innocent systolic murmur, venous hum, bicuspid aortic valve, and atrial septal defect out of my top six. Ventricular septal defect and patent ductus arteriosus remain in the same order. Considerably less likely are tetralogy of Fallot and pulmonary valve stenosis, in that order, followed by everything else.

Phase 3—I introduce myself to the mother and ask her to remove all clothes from the baby except the nappy and its cover. While she is doing this I ask her a few routine questions about pregnancy and family history. These are of considerably more value in making her feel at home than making a diagnosis. To be honest, the only question worth asking from a diagnostic point of view is whether the child has had any cyanotic spells. If the answer to this were yes Fallot's tetralogy would go to the top of the list. The answer is no. When the baby is undressed he turns out to look entirely healthy and acyanotic without breathing difficulty. This hardly affects the likelihood of ventricular septal defect, as the baby is as likely to appear normal with a ventricular septal defect as without. Patent ductus arteriosus becomes slightly less likely, but pulmonary valve stenosis overtakes tetralogy because most patients at this age who have tetralogy will be cyanosed while most who have pulmonary valve stenosis will not.

Phase 4—I feel the pulses. They are normal. If coarctation had been anywhere near the top of the table it would have dropped far down. As it is, patent ductus arteriosus drops to fourth place, as even fairly small ducts are associated with jerky pulses.

Phase 5—As this is a young baby I omit observing the jugular venous pulse for the time being and palpate the heart. There is a systolic thrill maximal in the third left intercostal space. This makes patent ductus arteriosus more unlikely still but moves ventricular septal defect a little further ahead of the rest.

Phase 6—I auscultate. There are no diastolic murmurs. The systolic murmur is of ejection type. There is an expiratory ejection click at the lower left sternal border, and pulmonary closure is delayed and quiet. Pulmonary valve stenosis moves to the top of the table, and everything else moves out of sight.

Note that the diagnosis has been achieved with parsimony yet without generating or testing a single hypothesis. The limitations of short term memory are dealt with by considering in detail only the top of the league table. A cross sectional echocardiogram is now ordered with a request for Doppler interrogation of the jet through the pulmonary valve to estimate the severity of the pulmonary stenosis. If the estimated gradient is less than 30 mm Hg we will simply follow up the patient. If it is above 30 mm Hg and there is no associated atrial septal defect the child will go for cardiac catheterisation and balloon valvuloplasty. If there is an atrial septal defect then the child will be referred for surgery without cardiac catheterisation. Thus the purpose of cross sectional echocardiography is primarily to help decision making. A secondary objective is to test the hypothesis that the patient has pulmonary valve stenosis without appreciable associated lesions.

The example given is typical of children of this age except that neither a chest x ray nor an electrocardiogram was required. If they had been performed they would simply have been regarded as phases 7 and 8, each requiring reassessment of the league table of probabilities.

Bayesian diagnosis

The diagnostic process will now be followed through mathematically. Let D_1, D_2 . . . D_n represent all n possible mutually exclusive diagnoses present. Then $P(D_1)$, $P(D_2)$ . . . $P(D_n)$ are the probabilities of diagnoses D_1, D_2, and so on. Table I gives the translations of D_1 to D_8. These probabilities correspond to population incidences of diagnoses and total 1. Each $P(D)$ is known as a prior probability, as it is a probability assessed before obtaining any further information.

At each phase of the investigation a clue to the diagnosis is given, which may be the answer to a question, the result of examining, say, the pulse, or the result of a laboratory test. The clue may be single (for example, the age of the patient) or composite (for example, the result of auscultation, which includes analysis of murmurs and sounds).

The first clue is that the patient has been referred to me, which

Table 1—Translation of diagnostic notation

D_1	Innocent systolic murmur
D_2	Venous hum
D_3	Bicuspid aortic valve
D_4	Ventricular septal defect
D_5	Atrial septal defect
D_6	Patent ductus arteriosus
D_7	Tetralogy of Fallot
D_8	Pulmonary valve stenosis

45

makes it much more likely that the child has heart disease. The probability of each diagnosis now becomes a conditional probability, also known in this case as a posterior probability because it represents the probability after the clue has been given. It is represented by $P(D_1|C_1)$, $P(D_2|C_1 \ldots P(D_n|C_1)$. C_1 is clue one. The vertical line is translated as "given that." It is rather unlikely that the conditional probability will be the same as the prior probability. For example, $P(D_7)$, the population incidence of tetralogy of Fallot, is around $0 \cdot 0007$. $P(D_7|C_1)$, the probability that the child has tetralogy given that he has been referred to me, is $0 \cdot 05$. $P(D_1|C_1)$, the probability that the child has an innocent systolic murmur, given that he has been referred to me, is $0 \cdot 4$. These conditional probabilities are simplest obtained by looking at all outpatients referred to me over the past five years, counting the types of diagnoses, and dividing by the number of new patients seen.

The second clue is that the baby is 3 months old. The conditional probability of D_1, innocent systolic murmur, now becomes $P(D_1|C_1$ and $C_2)$, which is $0 \cdot 05$, because referring doctors usually adopt a "wait and see" strategy at this age in fit patients who probably have innocent systolic murmurs. On the other hand, $P(D_4|C_1$ and $C_2)$ (ventricular septal defect) becomes $0 \cdot 35$, $P(D_5|C_1$ and $C_2)$ (atrial septal defect) becomes $0 \cdot 3$, $P(D_7|C_1$ and $C_2)$ (tetralogy) becomes $0 \cdot 15$, and $P(D_8|C_1$ and $C_2)$ (pulmonary valve stenosis) becomes $0 \cdot 08$. These figures are rounded off for simplicity. Again, they are best obtained by counting previously referred outpatients, this time stratifying according to age. Note how critically these probabilities depend on the nature of my referral practice. They differ widely from the probabilities that would apply to a general practitioner or a consultant paediatrician.

From local peculiarity to recorded cases

We now want to move on, however, from the peculiarities of the local situation to the point at which we can use information gleaned from the medical reports. To simplify matters we first note that at each phase of the analysis except the first the posterior probability for the previous stage becomes the prior probability for this one. Thus we may write $P(D_1\star) = P(D_1|C_1$ and $C_2)$, $P(D_2\star) = P(D_2|C_1$ and $C_2)$, and so on.

Clue 3 is that the child is acyanotic and having no difficulty in breathing. What we wish to know is $P(D^\star|C_3)$ for each diagnosis—for example, the probability that the child has a ventricular septal defect given that he looks normal. Unfortunately, textbooks and original articles are not usually written in such a way as to provide this information, because it requires, in effect, a chapter entitled "Acyanotic. No respiratory distress." Such a chapter heading would not even appear in a book on differential diagnosis. To be sure, such a book would contain a chapter headed "Cyanosis," but it can almost be guaranteed that all this chapter would contain is a list of diseases, whereas we want a probability. What we may find is a chapter headed "Ventricular septal defect," and with a bit of luck we can extract from this $P(C_3|D_4^\star)$, the probability that a child is acyanotic and in no distress given that he has a ventricular septal defect, is 3 months old, and has been referred to a consultant paediatric cardiologist (strictly speaking $D_4^\star$ refers to this paediatric cardiologist, but we have to assume unless there is good evidence to the contrary that the man who wrote the book is seeing the same kinds of patients as we are).

Is $P(C_3|D_4^\star)$ of any use to us? Not without Thomas Bayes, for his theorem allows us to calculate $P(D_4^\star|C_3)$ from $P(C_3|D_4^\star)$.

For the general diagnosis D and the general clue C:
$$P(D|C)=P(C|D)\cdot P(D)/(P(C|D)\cdot P(D)+P(C|\bar{D})\cdot P(\bar{D})).$$

$\bar{D}$, known as the complement of D, indicates the absence of that diagnosis. Now $P(C|\bar{D}\cdot P(\bar{D})$ is simply the sum of the products $(P(C|D_i)\cdot P(D_i))$, where the set of D_i consists of all mutually exclusive and exhaustive diagnoses apart from the one under consideration. $P(\bar{D})=1\text{-}P(D)$. Thus we may calculate $P(C|D)$ for each of five diagnoses, the four favourites and "everything else," to obtain the third column in table II. Each $P(C|\bar{D})$ corresponds to the false positive rate of a test for that diagnosis that is regarded as being positive in the absence of cyanosis or respiratory distress. It may be shown that the denominator in Bayes's expression is equal to $P(C)$, a result we shall use later.

For ventricular septal defect $P(C_3|D_4^\star)$ is 0.5 and $P(C_3|\bar{D}_4^\star)$ is 0.54.

$P(D_4^\star|C_3)=(0.5\times0.35)/((0.5\times0.35)+(0.54\times0.65))$, which gives the probability that the child has a ventricular septal defect, given that there is no cyanosis or respiratory distress. This is 0.35. The fourth column in table II show the posterior probabilities for the five diagnoses. Note that the probability of ventricular septal defect has remained unchanged, while patent ductus arteriosus has become less probable as a result of this observation. Pulmonary valve stenosis has

Table 2—*Bayes's theorem applied to congenital heart disease. Note that probabilities in first and fourth columns total 1, whereas probabilities in second and third columns do not*

Disease	$P(D^\star)$	$P(C_3|D^\star)$	$P(C_3|\bar{D}^\star)$	$P(D^\star|C_3)$
Ventricular septal defect (D_4)	0·35	0·50	0·54	0·35
Patent ductus arteriosus (D_6)	0·30	0·40	0·58	0·23
Tetralogy of Fallot (D_7)	0·15	0·30	0·56	0·09
Pulmonary valve stenosis (D_8)	0·08	0·90	0·49	0·14
Everything else	0·12	0·95	0·47	0·22

$P(D^\star)$=Probability that diagnosis $D^\star$ is correct.
$P(C_3|D^\star)$=Probability that child does not have cyanosis or respiratory distress given that diagnosis $D^\star$ is correct.
$P(C_3|\bar{D}^\star)$=Probability that child does not have cyanosis or respiratory distress given that diagnosis $D^\star$ is incorrect.
$P(D^\star|C_3)$=Probability that diagnosis $D^\star$ is correct given that child does not have cyanosis or respiratory distress.

edged ahead of tetralogy of Fallot, as expected. The alert reader will have observed that it is possible to calculate the figures in the fourth column of table II directly from those in the first and second columns without calculating the values in the third column.

At each stage of the diagnosis these probabilities are revised until pulmonary stenosis emerges as a clear favourite. Thus we see that the diagnostic process originally described bears a remarkably close resemblance to successive applications of Bayes's theorem, the differences being that ranked probabilities rather than actual probabilities are used and no calculations are consciously made. It seems likely, however, that the reordering of ranked probabilities occurs as a result of intuitive mathematics. This interpretation is strengthened when it is appreciated that Bayes's theorem can be rewritten as: posterior odds=prior odds×likelihood ratio, where prior odds are the ratio between the probability of a diagnosis and the probability of its complement and likelihood ratio is the ratio of the probability of a positive clue in the presence and absence of the diagnosis.

Thus in the above example the prior odds on pulmonary valve stenosis were 0·08/0·92—that is, 0·087. The likelihood ratio was 0·9/0·49—that is, 1·84. The posterior odds rise to 0·087×1·84—that is, 0·16. In gambling terms the odds against pulmonary valve stenosis have shortened from 11 to 1 (11 is the reciprocal of 0·087) to 6 to 1. Gambling on horses would be a great deal less popular were not punters confident of their intuitive ability to adjust gambling odds in the light of new information. One further refinement of this application is to take the natural logarithm of the likelihood ratio and call this "the weight of evidence."[31][32]

Bayes's theorem

A probabilistic approach is helpful not only because it models what some clinicians do but, even more importantly, it also illuminates issues that are not at all clear to many otherwise extremely competent diagnosticians. The most striking of these issues is the way in which prior probabilities can affect the usefulness of a test.

A good example is the hyperoxic test for congenital heart disease in neonates who seem to be cyanosed. This consists of letting the baby breathe 100% oxygen for 10 minutes and then measuring the systemic arterial oxygen pressure.[33] Table III shows the results. In figure 1 (a) these have been drawn as a probability tree. We take first the left hand tree. Here the prior probabilities of cyanotic heart disease, acyanotic heart disease, and lung disease have been obtained by dividing the column total of table III by the grand total. These probabilities are inserted on the top three branches of the tree. Each of these forks into two, depending on whether the $Po_2 > 150$ mm Hg or $\leqslant 150$ mm Hg. These branches are labelled with the conditional probability calculated by dividing the numbers in each cell of table III by the column total (for example, $p(>150|\text{cyanotic} = 2/109 = 0.02$). Notice that the probabilities on the branches of the tree are conditional on the events above them.

As has already been pointed out, the conditional probabilities on

Table 3—Results of hyperoxic test for congenital heart disease[33]

	Congenital heart disease			
	Cyanotic	Acyanotic	Lung disease	Total
Po_2 (mm Hg):				
>150	2	153	7	162
≤150	107	0	16	123
Total	109	153	23	285

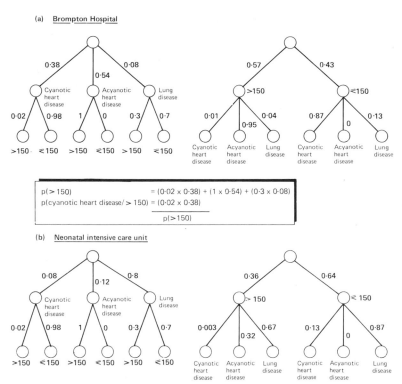

FIG 1—(a) Probability trees corresponding to results of hyperoxic test at specialist referral centre for paediatric cardiology. Equations show calculation of posterior probabilities for inversion of the probability tree. (b) Probability trees corresponding to results of hyperoxic test at neonatal intensive care unit.

this tree are not particularly useful in diagnosis, but they are important in that we may be fairly sure that if the same test is carried out in a different environment the same conditional probabilities will emerge. In other words, the sensitivity and selectivity of the test are reasonably robust.

To obtain diagnostic information we need to invert the network, as shown in the right hand tree of figure 1 (a), to obtain probabilities conditional on the result of the test rather than on the type of disorder present. This network has two prior probabilities, corresponding to the two possible results, and three branches for each, representing the diseases. It can be obtained from table III by dividing the row totals by the grand totals to give the prior probabilities and numbers in each cell by row totals to give conditional probabilities. Using Bayes's theorem

Table 4—Posterior probabilities of diagnoses based on results of hyperoxic test

	Congenital heart disease		
	Cyanotic	Acyanotic	Lung disease
pO$_2$>150 mm Hg:			
Brompton	0·01	0·95	0·04
Neonatal intensive care unit	0·003	0·32	0·67
pO$_2$≤150 mm Hg:			
Brompton	0·87	0	0·13
Neonatal intensive care unit	0·13	0	0·87

will give the same result. It is possible to apply this directly to the network by observing that joint probabilities (for example p(>150 and cyanotic)) are obtained by multiplying together the probabilities on the pathways through cyanotic and >150. To obtain p(>150) we sum the joint probabilities involving >150, which amounts to calculating the denominator in Bayes's theorem. Any conditional probability (for example, p(cyanotic|>150) is then calculated by dividing the numerator in Bayes's equation (for example, p(cyanotic and >150) by the denominator.

Table IV shows the posterior probabilities for the Brompton Hospital (a specialist centre for paediatric cardiology and cardiac surgery). The hyperoxic test is seen to be very useful in that if the Po$_2$ >150 mm Hg the diagnosis is almost certainly acyanotic heart disease and highly unlikely to be cyanotic heart disease. If, on the other hand, the Po$_2$ ≤150 mm Hg cyanotic heart disease is highly likely (p=0·87).

Now let us consider the performance of this test in a typical neonatal intensive care unit, where the cause of cyanosis in 80% of cases is lung disease. The left hand network of figure 1 (*b*) has been calculated on the assumption that cyanotic and non-cyanotic infants are distributed as for the specialist centre but make up only 20% of the whole. The probabilities conditional on the diagnosis are assumed to be the same as at the specialist centre for reasons already given. This network has then been inverted as already described to obtain the right hand network, and the probabilities conditional on the result of the test have been transferred to table IV. Observe that whatever the Po$_2$ the likeliest diagnosis is lung disease. Why? Because the prior probability of lung disease is so high. What is a good test in a specialist referral centre is really of no use in a neonatal intensive care unit.

The second great advantage of a probabilistic approach to diagnosis is that with little extra computational effort it can be extended into decision theory to allow the cost of an investigation to be traded off against the information it provides, thus increasing parsimony. Similarly, a decision analysis approach allows us to decide how certain we have to be about a particular diagnosis before we apply treatment on the assumption that the diagnosis is correct. As decision theory will be covered later in this series no more will be said now, but interested readers should refer to Weinstein *et al*[34] and Macartney *et al*.[35]

The mathematical foundation of Bayes's theorem makes it an ideal computer model; probably the most successful diagnosis program yet devised for a computer was an early application of Bayes's theorem to the acute abdomen.[36] The computer was shown to be better than clinicians in making the diagnosis. Equally important was the fact that implementing the computerised system improved clinicians' performances by showing which clues were most helpful in discriminating diseases.[37] Other Bayesian systems have been described for congenital heart disease,[38] classification of stroke,[39] identifying those who will attempt suicide,[40] diagnosing solitary pulmonary nodules,[41] and dyspepsia.[42]

If the "weight of evidence" as defined above is multiplied by 100 and rounded off for convenience a rather simple means of summing the weights of evidence for and against a particular diagnosis and working back to the probability of that diagnosis can be obtained.[15] The two advantages of this approach are, firstly, that it allows statistical diagnosis without a computer once the weights of evidence have been calculated and, secondly, that if a computer is used the output consists of a list of weights of evidence that are intuitively easily understood by the clinician. Thus the machine "explains" how it has come to a particular diagnosis. Approaches by artificial intelligence to diagnosis have always emphasised how important explanation is[43] and have criticised statistical methods for their failure to explain themselves.[44]

One objection often raised to such uses of Bayes's theorem is that they assume the conditional independence of clues—that is, that the probability of a given clue in the presence of disease remains the same regardless of the presence or absence of all the other clues. Clearly this does not always apply. The probability of cyanosis given tetralogy of Fallot and finger clubbing is not the same as that given tetralogy without finger clubbing, as finger clubbing and cyanosis are almost always associated beyond the age of 1 year. It is possible to apply

Bayes's theorem without assuming conditional independence,[45] but the best way of dealing with the lack of conditional independence is to use multivariate analysis, as described below.

As a model of clinical behaviour a Bayesian approach has been shown to be as plausible as the hypotheticodeductive, certainly in those cases where the history is unimportant. The fact that the question of transferability—that is, whether the system developed in one environment will work in another—has been raised so often in the context of Bayesian systems[39 46] seems to me to be a strength of the Bayesian approach rather than a weakness, as however diseases are diagnosed (unless by pathognomic clues, which are rare) prior probabilities matter, and Bayes's theorem shows why.

Alternative statistical models allowing for conditional dependence

One solution to the problem of dependence is linear discriminant function analysis, shown in figure 2. Figure 2 (a) shows the distribution of a continuous variable F_1 between two categories of patient, each with one of two diagnoses. Values of F_1 are displayed on a one dimensional line. A line at right angles intersects this line at a point whose position is calculated to maximise separation of the values of F_1 for the two sets of patients, but there is considerable overlap.

A second continuous variable F_2 is added to the model at right angles to F_1; this allows the results to be displayed on a two dimensional plane (fig 2 (b)). The two disease spaces are now separated by a discriminant line, again calculated to maximise separation of the two sets of patients. Overlap has been reduced but is still present.

Now F_3 is introduced at right angles to F_1 and F_2. The observations now occupy a three dimensional space separated by a two dimensional plane (fig 2 (c)). Now complete separation of the two diagnoses has been achieved. Furthermore (as with the first two stages), posterior probabilities for a single patient can be calculated from the distance between the point corresponding to that patient and the discriminant plane.

Three dimensions is as much as the human mind can imagine, but in mathematics there is no limit to the number of dimensions and therefore no problem in conceiving a 31 dimensional space separated into two (or more) components by a 30 dimensional space. Conditional dependence is allowed for, as it alters the weights of the discriminant variables in the model.

Linear discriminant function analysis therefore provides a powerful method of computer assisted diagnosis.[47] Its use is commonly facilitated by stepwise procedures that fit first the best discriminating feature, then allow for this and fit the next best discriminator, and so on. By this means a parsimonious set of relatively few discriminators may be selected. Forward stepwise regression does not, however, necessarily pick the best set of predictors. Such a procedure does not attempt to model human diagnostic logic, although it can be explained in a way that makes sense to most clinicians.

One disadvantage of linear discriminant function analysis is that the calculation of posterior probabilities is not all that simple.[48] Multiple logistic regression has the advantage that, given the set of discriminators and their weights, the likelihood ratio is easily calculated. Another possibility is non-parametric discriminant analysis.[49]

The ultimate in statistical diagnosis is to make no prior assumptions about diagnostic categories but to let the data speak for themselves.

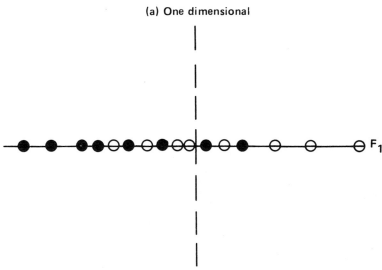

(a) One dimensional

Fig 2a

FIG 2—(a) Discriminant function analysis in one dimension. (b) Discriminant function analysis in two dimensions. (c) Discriminant function analysis in three dimensions.

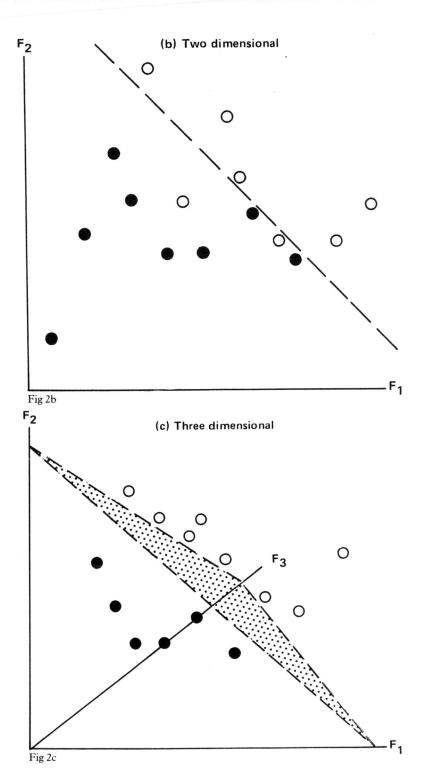

(b) Two dimensional

Fig 2b

(c) Three dimensional

Fig 2c

This corresponds to syndromic diagnosis by computer. For obvious reasons this approach has been mostly applied to the diagnosis of mental illness, in which there is considerable doubt about the validity of traditional diagnostic categories. On the whole, however, these multivariate methods (factor and cluster analysis) have proved to be disappointing.[1]

Conclusions

No explanation of human diagnostic logic so far conceived has been entirely satisfactory, though study of the alternative models is extremely instructive. Similarly, no method of diagnosis helped by computers has been shown consistently to be superior to all others. This is an exciting field of research precisely because it is so wide open. The validation of approaches by artificial intelligence to diagnosis has been particularly scanty—either non-existent or based on fewer than 20 patients. It is essential that comparisons of alternative diagnostic aids[44 50-52] should be carried out as stringently as are those at present for new therapeutic aids such as drugs.

1 Kendell RE. *The role of diagnosis in psychiatry.* Oxford: Blackwell, 1975.
2 Wulff HR. *Rational diagnosis and treatment. An introduction to clinical decision-making.* 2nd ed. Oxford: Blackwell, 1981.
3 Scadding JG. Diagnosis: the clinician and the computer. *Lancet* 1967;ii:877-82.
4 Campbell EJM. The science of diagnosis. In: Phillips CI, Wolfe JN, eds. *Clinical practice and economics.* London: Pitman Publishing, 1977:101-12.
5 Okada M, Maruyama N, Kanda T, Shirakawa K, Katagiri T. Medical data base system with an ability of automated diagnosis. *Comput Programs Biomed* 1977;7:163-70.
6 Winter RM, Baraitser M, Douglas JM. A computerised data base for the diagnosis of rare dysmorphic syndromes. *J Med Genet* 1984;21:121-3.
7 Williams BT. *Computer aids to clinical decisions.* Vols I and II. Florida: CRC Press, 1982.
8 Bleich HL. Computer-based consultation: electrolyte and acid-base disorders. *Am J Med* 1972;53:285-91.
9 Vastola EF. Assign: an automated screening system in general neurology. *Comput Biol Med* 1973;3:107-9.
10 Davis R, King J. An overview of production systems. In: Elcock E, Michie D, eds. *Machine intelligence.* New York: Wiley, 1976:300-32.
11 Waterman D, Hayes-Roth F. An overview of pattern-directed inference systems. In: Waterman D, Hayes-Roth F, eds. *Pattern directed inference systems.* London: Academic Press, 1978: 3-22.
12 Weiss S, Kulikowski C, Safir A. Glaucoma consultation by computer. *Comput Biol Med* 1978;8:25-40.
13 Reggia JA. A production rule system for neurological localisation. In: *Proceedings of second annual symposium of computer applications to medical care, New York.* New York: IEEE, 1978:254-60.
14 Davis R, Buchanan B, Shortliffe E. Production rules as a representation for a knowledge-based consultation program. *Artificial Intelligence* 1977;8:15-45.

15 Spiegelhalter DJ, Knill-Jones RP. Statistical and knowledge-based approaches to clinical decision-support systems, with an application to gastroenterology. *Journal of Royal Statistical Society A* 1984;**147**(Pt 1):35-77.
16 Inhelder B, Piaget J. *The growth of logical thinking from childhood to adolescence*. London: Routledge & Kegan Paul, 1958.
17 Campbell EJM. Basic science, science and medical education. *Lancet* 1976;i:134-6.
18 Campbell EJM. Clinical science. *Clinical Science and Molecular Medicine* 1976;**51**:1-7.
19 Magee B. *Popper*. London: Woburn Press, 1974.
20 Elstein AS, Shulman LS, Sprafka SA. *Medical problem solving: an analysis of clinical reasoning*. Cambridge, Massachussetts: Harvard University Press, 1978.
21 Kassirer JP, Gorry GA. Clinical problem solving. A behavioural analysis. *Ann Intern Med* 1978;**89**:245-55.
22 Medawar PB. *Induction and intuition in scientific thought*. London: Methuen 1969.
23 Menninger K. *The vital balance: the life process in mental health and illness*. New York: Viking Press 1963.
24 Cutler P. *Problem solving in clinical medicine. From data to diagnosis*. 2nd ed. Baltimore: Williams & Wilkins, 1985.
25 Elstein AS, Kagan N, Shulman LS, Jason H, Loupe M. Methods and theory in the study of medical enquiry. *J Med Educ* 1972;**47**:85-92.
26 Reggia JA, Tuhrim S. An overview of methods for computer-assisted medical decision making. In: Reggia JA, Tuhrim S, eds. *Computer-assisted medical decision making*. New York: Springer-Verlag, 1985:3-45.
27 Pauker SG, Gorry GA, Kassirer JP, Schwartz WB. Towards the simulation of clinical cognition: taking a present illness by computer. *Am J Med* 1976;**60**:981-96.
28 Reggia JA, Nau DS, Wang PY. Diagnostic expert systems based on a set covering model. *International Journal of Man-Machine Studies* 1983;**19**:437-60.
29 Miller RA, Pople HE, Jr, Myers JD. INTERNIST-1. An experimental computer-based diagnostic consultant for general internal medicine. *N Engl J Med* 1982;**307**:468-76.
30 Pople HE. Heuristic methods for imposing structure on ill structured problems: the structuring of medical diagnosis. In: Szolovitz P, ed. *Artificial intelligence in medicine*. Colorado: Westview Press, 1982: 119-85.
31 Good IJ. Weight of evidence, corroboration, explanatory power, information and the utility of experiments. *J R Statist Soc* 1960;**22**(B):319-31.
32 Good IJ, Card WI. The diagnostic process with special reference to errors. *Methods Inf Med* 1971;**10**:176-88.
33 Jones RWA, Baumer JH, Joseph MC, Shinebourne EA. Arterial oxygen tension and response to oxygen breathing in differential diagnosis of congenital heart disease in infancy. *Arch Dis Child* 1976;**51**:667-73.
34 Weinstein MC, Fineberg HV, Elstein AS, et al. *Clinical decision analysis*. Philadelphia: WB Saunders, 1980.
35 Macartney FJ, Douglas J, Spiegelhalter D. To catheterise or not to catheterise? An approach based on decision theory. *Br Heart J* 1984;**51**:330-8.
36 De Dombal FT, Leaper DJ, Staniland JR, McCann AP, Horrocks JC. Computer-aided diagnosis of acute abdominal pain. *Br Med J* 1972;ii:9-13.
37 De Dombal FT, Leaper DJ, Horrocks JC, Staniland JR, McCann AP. Human and computer aided diagnosis of abdominal pain: further report with emphasis on performance of clinicians. *Br Med J* 1974;i:376-80.
38 Warner HR, Toronto AF, Veasy LG, Stephenson RS. A mathematical approach to medical diagnosis: application to congenital heart disease. *JAMA* 1961;**177**:177-83.
39 Zagoria R, Reggia J. Transferability of medical decision support systems based on Bayesian classification. *Med Decis Making* 1983;**3**:501-9.
40 Gustafson DH, Greist JH, Stauss FF, Erdman H, Laughren T. A probabilistic system for identifying suicide attemptors. *Comput Biomed Res* 1977;**10**:83-9.
41 Templeton AW, Jansen C, Lehr JL, Hufft R. Solitary pulmonary lesions. Computer-aided differential diagnosis and evaluation of mathematical methods. *Radiology* 1967;**89**:605-13.
42 Horrocks JC, De Dombal FT. Computer aided diagnosis of "dyspepsia." *American Journal of Digestive Diseases* 1975;**20**:397-406.
43 Teach RL, Shortliffe EH. An analysis of physician attitudes regarding computer-based clinical consultation systems. *Comput Biomed Res* 1981;**14**:542-58.
44 Fox J, Barber D, Bardhan KD. Alternative to Bayes? A quantitative comparison with rule-based diagnostic inference. *Methods Inf Med* 1980;**19**:210-5.

57

45 Fryback DG. Bayes' theorem and conditional non-independence of data in medical diagnosis. *Comput Biomed Res* 1978;**11**:423-34.
46 Zoltie N, Horrocks JC, De Dombal FT. Computer-assisted diagnosis of dyspepsia—report on transferability of a system, with emphasis on early diagnosis of gastric cancer. *Methods Inf Med* 1977;**16**:89-92.
47 Macartney FJ, Rees PG, Daly K, *et al*. Angiocardiographic appearances of atrioventricular defects with particular reference to distinction of ostium primum atrial septal defect from common atrioventricular orifice. *Br Heart J* 1979;**42**:640-56.
48 Lachenbruch PA. Evaluating a discriminant function. In: Lachenbruch PA, ed. *Discriminant analysis*. New York: Macmillan, 1975:25-39.
49 Habbema JDF, Gelpke GJ. A computer program for selection of variables in diagnostic and prognostic problems. *Comput Programs Biomed* 1981;**13**:251-70.
50 Croft DJ, Machol RE. Mathematical methods in medical diagnosis. *Ann Biomed Eng* 1974;**2**: 69-89.
51 Nordyke RA, Kulikowski CA, Kulikowski CW. A comparison of methods for the automated diagnosis of thyroid dysfunction. *Comput Biomed Res* 1971;**4**:374-89.
52 Fleiss JL, Spitzer RL, Cohen J, Endicott J. Three computer diagnosis methods compared. *Arch Gen Psychiatry* 1972;**27**:643-9.

Diagnostic systems as an aid to clinical decision making

R P KNILL-JONES

My contribution to this series on logic in medicine aims to carry the theme of "diagnostic logic" discussed by Macartney in the previous chapter[1] further in the direction of clinical decision making. The example of dyspepsia has been chosen, partly because it has long been one of my special interests; the underlying principles exemplified are, however, applicable to many other clinical problems.

Dyspepsia diagnosis

However defined, dyspepsia is a common condition that accounts for a considerable proportion of consultations in general practice, referrals to hospital, and working days lost to illness. Diagnosis is often difficult and negative results of investigations common,[2] which leads to many patients having the symptoms but no evidence of an organic cause for them. An accurate history is therefore essential, yet one may not be taken because of lack of time, the easy availability of investigations such as endoscopy (which seems sometimes to be used as an alternative to a properly taken history), or a simple failure to appreciate the discriminating value of standardised questions. Several solutions to this problem have been explored, including the use of standard forms[3] that can be entered on a computer,[4] automated history taking,[5 6] which can be used as a decision aid,[7 8] and simple weighting systems for symptoms.[9 10]

All these solutions aim to reduce the diagnostic uncertainty of the doctor so that more rational therapeutic, investigative, and referral procedures develop. Diagnostic uncertainty about patients who have dyspepsia is high in general practice and is probably equally high among junior hospital staff; despite such uncertainty, there is little teaching about which are the best questions to ask—that is, which are the Popperian searchlights alluded to by Macartney.

What is required is a simple screening system that minimises unnecessary referrals and negative results of investigations. The development of such a system has many similarities to problems in other clinical specialties. For example, in the assessment of risk for ischaemic heart disease the use of weights (or scores) for each factor is becoming widespread.[11] In this instance the approach is a practical one for assessing risk, and it can help patients to reduce their own risk factors. In dyspepsia a similar approach should lead to better use of existing resources and in particular improve the overall management of patients when care is shared between the general practitioner and the hospital based specialist.

This paper shows first how a simple weighting system for symptoms can be devised, given some carefully collected data. The method is clearly related to that described by Macartney but is expressed in a different way. For application in clinical practice this process has been partly automated: a computer asks the relevant questions of the patient and prints the results as a summary; this is effectively a screening process indicating which patients require referral and why, and, for those who do not indicating appropriate management to be carried out in general practice.

Weighting of symptoms

There are several steps in the process of developing weights for symptoms.

(1) Defining the population of patients

The first step is to define the population of interest. In this example I have used a wide definition of dyspepsia which includes many patients with non-acute gastrointestinal symptoms. This broad definition reflects the poor localisation of symptoms within the gastrointestinal tract and is as follows: "Episodic, persistent, or recurrent abdominal pain or discomfort or any other symptoms referrable to the alimentary tract except for rectal bleeding and jaundice as the main symptom."

(2) Defining (relevant) symptoms

The second step is to define the symptoms relevant to dyspepsia. This is much more important than is commonly realised, the underlying assumption being that we all know what is meant by simple terms such as "flatulence" and "nausea." If colleagues are asked to write down definitions, however, there are big differences, not only in length but also in meaning. For example, "flatulence" to 19 of 40 gastroenterologists meant passing wind upwards, to seven passing wind through the rectum, and to 11 passing wind in either direction.[12]

Thus the evidence that we can discard explicit definitions in favour of our implicit ones is not good. We have to agree on some kind of definition of a symptom and try to stick to it when collecting data. Clinicians are not entirely comfortable with this concept, but epidemiologists are, having learnt to live with it.

In our studies on dyspepsia definitions have been given for every symptom on the form used for collecting data; though this does not completely remove inconsistencies among observers,[12] it does seem to reduce them. For example, the written definition we have used for flatulence is: "The patient brings up what he regards as an excessive amount of wind," while for nausea the patient feels "sick without actually being sick." By contrast, the form widely used for assessing acute pain in the abdomen does not contain definitions of each term used; definitions, however, are now available on separate sheets when required.[13] Perhaps surgeons have more consistent implicit definitions than physicians?

Some 1200 patients have now been seen in the study of dyspepsia at the Southern General Hospital in Glasgow, and, of these, nearly half were aged under 40 at the time of presentation, just over half having had symptoms for less than two years. The commonest presenting symptom was abdominal pain or discomfort (64%), the next commonest being vomiting and diarrhoea (7% each) and heartburn (5%). On direct questioning 87% of patients agreed that they had had some abdominal pain or discomfort, even if in a quarter it had not been their presenting symptom. One fifth of all our patients had had at least one episode of pain sufficiently severe to call in a doctor as an emergency or to attend an accident and emergency department. Few had a final diagnosis normally recognised as causing an "acute abdomen." Many must therefore have been patients who when presenting with acute pain were discharged with a diagnosis of "non-specific abdominal pain," a term used for 34% of presentations in a recent multicentre study.[4] There are many definable and treatable diagnoses in this heterogeneous group, which can be somewhat misleadingly used as a diagnostic dustbin.

These first two steps allow us to define an area of interest and collect data in a reasonably reproducible way. An analysis of these data allows a population of patients to be described simply—giving for example, the prevalence of symptoms in a hospital clinic, as was done briefly in the preceding paragraph.

(3) Defining the diagnosis

The third step is to define the diagnosis. To find out which symptoms are diagnostic rather than descriptive it is clearly essential to obtain a "final diagnosis" for every patient. This is not particularly easy for dyspepsia. Although we could not provide any diagnosis at all in only 2% of our patients (usually because of failure of follow up), we found it difficult to be absolutely certain about a final diagnosis on many occasions. Furthermore, there is always some residual uncertainty about whether a patient's symptoms are in fact due to the particular diagnosis with which he has been labelled, given the poor specificity of symptoms arising from the gastrointestinal tract. This also makes an algorithmic approach inherently implausible, at least for most gastrointestinal disease.

As a result of this uncertainty, early in the study it proved to be necessary, firstly, to allow the possibility of there being more than one gastrointestinal diagnosis in a patient, and, secondly, to indicate for each final diagnosis given whether it was certain, probable, or possible. This reflected the completeness of follow up and the adequacy of investigation. For instance, a patient who had a duodenal ulcer that was seen clearly at endoscopy and noted then as being present without any doubt and was confirmed after a barium meal would have a "certain" final diagnosis of a duodenal ulcer. If in addition the patient had several symptoms of irritable bowel syndrome, sufficient to fit a pattern about which there was considerable agreement,[14][15] then he would have a second diagnosis of irritable bowel syndrome. The order in which the diagnoses were given would reflect the clinician's opinion on which was the more important condition for that patient. About one third of our patients had a second diagnosis.

Recording the final diagnosis in this way is important for developing weights for symptoms. In an analysis of the symptoms of patients who have a duodenal ulcer the patients can be selected according to whether they have one or more than one final diagnosis. If the weights of the symptoms seem to be similar then both groups could be combined; if not then care would be necessary in selecting both patients and symptoms.

The same procedure can be applied to the certainty of final diagnosis. If patients who have a certain final diagnosis of duodenal ulcer are symptomatically similar to those who have a probable diagnosis both groups can be included when calculating symptom weights.

Table 1 shows the broad groupings of the final diagnoses in the first 1200 patients in our study. No final diagnosis could be made in 2%, who were excluded. About one quarter of all the patients had duodenal ulcer disease, and a further 74 (6%) had gastric ulcer. Another quarter had non-organic dyspepsia or functional dyspepsia,

Table 1—Broad disease classification (primary diagnosis) of cases of dyspepsia seen at Southern General Hospital, Glasgow

	No (%) of patients	
Uncomplicated oesophageal disease	45	(4)
Severe oesophageal disease	63	(5)
Gastric ulcer	74	(6)
Carcinoma of stomach	32	(3)
Duodenal ulcer disease	330	(27)
Cholelithiasis	50	(4)
Irritable bowel syndrome	177	(15)
Non-organic dyspepsia	294	(25)
Alcohol related dyspepsia	48	(4)
Organic bowel disease, undiagnosed	87	(7)
Total	1200 (100)	

and to these some might wish to add the 177 patients (15%) who had irritable bowel syndrome. The final diagnosis was certain in about 60% of the patients who had duodenal ulcer, nearly 81% of the patients who had gastric ulcer, about 40% of those who had non-organic dyspepsia, and half of the patients who had a primary diagnosis of irritable bowel syndrome.

(4) Evaluating the weights of symptoms numerically

There have been many reported examples of the use of Bayes's theorem to produce a diagnostic aid of some kind—for example, in jaundice[16][17] and in the very different problem of prognosis after head injury.[18] In some of these problems the presentation of the basic method has been altered so that clinicians are given a series of weights of symptoms that can be printed on a simple card and added up according to which symptoms the patient has. Thus the fourth step, the data on patients having been obtained and their problems finally diagnosed, is to analyse the data in such a way as to obtain the weights of symptoms.

The most successful example of this has been for jaundice, where the COMIK group in Copenhagen have described and tested a pocket chart based on a scoring system derived from Bayes's theorem.[19] This work developed from earlier work on jaundice by way of a careful comparison, carried out in 1980, of variation among observers in assessing symptoms.[20] Similar scoring systems have not yet been developed for the acutely painful abdomen, although several groups interested in the problem will probably produce one soon.

The assumption is, of course, that the explicit provision of weights for symptoms is better understood by clinicians than a little black box that calculates the probability of disease in the way that the classical applications of Bayes's theorem have done. Although there is no definite evidence to confirm this assumption, it does seem likely to be right.

To show how simple weightings for symptoms can be developed I shall show how such a system differentiates between two groups of patients presenting with dyspepsia, one with duodenal ulcer as the cause and the other with gastric ulcer as the cause. At this point you might like to consider carefully which symptoms might conceivably differentiate between these two conditions.

As encouragement one immediate suggestion is that it is well known for duodenal ulcers to be commoner in men and gastric ulcers to be commoner in women. Perhaps you would agree that men make up some 70% of the patients who have duodenal ulcer compared with only 35% of the patients who have gastric ulcer? A fairly obvious way of expressing the weight of this particular "symptom"—that is, the sex of the patient—is to divide 70 by 35 to give a ratio of 2. This means that a patient who has a duodenal ulcer is twice as likely to be a man than a patient who has a gastric ulcer. The ratio is also equivalent to the epidemiological idea of relative risk, and this natural ratio is also closely related to the well known concepts of sensitivity and specificity, which are normally applied to screening tests; the ratio is simply: sensitivity÷(1−specificity). This ratio is, of course, exactly the same as the likelihood ratio mentioned by Macartney.[1]

One way of thinking about the clinical consultation is to regard every question or investigation as a kind of screening test. Thus the apparent dissimilarity between the clinical consultation on the one hand and the assessment of screening tests on the other is not perhaps quite as great as it might at first seem.

The example taken below includes about 75% of our patients who had duodenal ulcer, excluding those who had multiple diagnoses or an uncertain diagnosis, and about 60% of our patients who had gastric ulcer, selected in the same way.

The actual figures from the study (table 2) show that there was a preponderance of men among the cases of duodenal ulcer—namely, 169 of 248 (68%)—compared with 17 of 43 cases of gastric ulcer (40%). If the dyspepsia sufferer is a man duodenal ulcer is therefore more likely, and this would naturally be expected to give a positive weight towards the diagnosis of duodenal ulcer. Using the example of the simple ratio given above we find that the actual ratio is 68/40, or 1.7.

To turn the ratio into a simple score that we can add up we now have to take the logarithm of this ratio (technically a likelihood ratio), because logarithms can be added rather than needing to be multiplied, thus simplifying the process. In this case the natural logarithm of the ratio is 0·531. Again to make it simple to use, this value is multiplied by 10 and rounded to allow us to quote some whole numbers as weights; in this case the weight to be applied in favour of duodenal ulcers for patients who are men is $10 \times 0·531 = 5$.

If, however, the patient in our clinic is a woman then a different weight has to be calculated. In this case the ratio is $32\% \div 60\% = 0·53$,

Table 2—*Crude weights for symptoms of duodenal ulcer and gastric ulcer, and effect of adjustment of crude scores by logistic determination. Crude weights were derived from available data for selected indicants and cases*

Symptom	Duodenal ulcer (n=248)	Gastric ulcer (n=43)	Crude weights	Adjusted weight (by logistic discrimination)	Standard error	Expected value of each question (for duodenal ulcer)
Men	169	17	5	3	1·3	0·1
Women	79	26	−6	−6	2·4	
Age (years):						
<26	43	1	18	18	3·7	4·0
26-40	82	5	10	8	1·4	
41-55	87	19	−2	−1	0·9	
>55	36	18	−10	−10	3·2	
Daily pain:						
Yes	21	11	−12	−11	4·1	0·8
No	214	27	3	2	0·6	
Effect of food on pain:						
Worse	44	11	−4	−6	2·9	0·2
Same	82	9	4	5	2·3	
Improved	104	17	0	−1	0·3	
Prior probability	0·85	0·15	17	20	1·8	

Weightings for symptoms given above are provisional and are being revised to take account of additional cases.

for which the logarithm is negative (-0.629). Multiplying by 10 gives us a score of -6.

The weights seem to be reasonably natural, in the sense that if the patient is a man we add some five points towards a diagnosis of duodenal ulcer and if the patient is a woman then we subtract six from the score for duodenal ulcer.

Table 2 gives the data and the corresponding weights for a few illustrative symptoms. The table shows that a further weight, reflecting the fact that duodenal ulcer is much more common than gastric ulcer, has to be added in. This final weight ($+17$) reflects the prior probability of disease and is specific to our clinic. To use the weights elsewhere other values can readily be substituted for our prior probability. The calculation of this weight proceeds exactly as before: thus the value of $+17$ in table II is derived from the ratio prior probability of duodenal ulcer/prior probability of gastric ulcer$=0.85/0.15=5.67$. The logarithm of $5.67 \times 10 = 17$ (to the nearest whole number).

The following two examples show how the scores are added up to form a total from which the probability can be derived. The calculations to convert a total score back to a probability of disease (technically a posterior probability) are shown in the next section.

Take a woman aged 30 who does not have daily pain and who finds that food makes the pain worse. Table 2 shows that in this case there are two negative scores (-6 for being a woman and -4 for food aggravation) that total -10 and three positive scores ($+10$ for age, $+3$ for no daily pain, and $+17$ for prior probability) that add up to $+30$, giving a net score of $+20$. Given that she has some kind of ulcer, this converts to a probability of this woman having a duodenal ulcer of 88% compared with her chances of having a gastric ulcer of 12%.

To take another example, if we had a woman aged 65 who had daily pain and symptoms suggesting that food made the pain worse then she would have a total score of -32, which, when combined with the prior probability score of $+17$, gives a total of -15, in turn converting to a probability of a duodenal ulcer of 18% and a much higher probability of a gastric ulcer of 82%.

The conversion of a patient's cumulative score to probability is straightforward. Remember to divide the score by 10 to reverse the previous step of multiplying the logarithm by 10. To take the first example above:

Cumulative score (T) $\qquad = 30 + (-10) = 20.$

$$\text{Probability of duodenal ulcer} = 1\cdot0 \div (\text{antilog } \tfrac{-T}{10} + 1\cdot0)$$
$$= 1\cdot0 \div (\text{antilog } (-2) + 1\cdot0)$$
$$= 1\cdot0 \div 1\cdot14$$
$$= 0\cdot88 \text{ or } 88\%.$$

This can be done more quickly by using a simple graph.[21]

(5) Logistic discrimination to adjust weights for dependence between symptoms

The fifth step required by this method reflects a well known statistical problem with Bayes's theorem: the assumption, in its basic form, of independence of symptoms within a class of diseases. For example, in a patient with jaundice it is clear that in biliary obstruction the symptom of passing dark urine is highly correlated with (or dependent on) another symptom—namely, passing pale stools. Thus these two symptoms are clearly not independent, though on occasions when only one of the two occurs without the other some diagnostic information might be obtained. The uncritical use of simple Bayes's theorem, which some authors have been known to describe as "idiot's Bayes," particularly in its blunderbuss form, leads to considerable problems in overestimating the probabilities of disease. This happens if many symptoms that are highly dependent on each other are included.

It is therefore necessary to find statistical ways of making an adjustment, and this can be done by several methods, the most appropriate of which seems to be logistic discrimination. (An extensive example of its application to dyspepsia is available.[10]). What this does is to reduce the weights of symptoms for those indicants that are dependent on, or correlated with, other indicants, thereby avoiding the resulting overestimation of probabilities. The effect of this is also shown in table II, which compares the crude weightings obtained earlier with the slightly reduced weightings obtained after adjustment by logistic discrimination. For this particular example the effects on the probabilities of disease for the two patients given in an earlier section are not very great. The first example had a combined score of 20 when crude weights were used, and this becomes 18 when adjusted weights are used, changing the probability of duodenal ulcer from 88% to 86%. In the second example the probability of duodenal ulcer changes from 18% to 21%.

You should not go away with the idea that adjustments to crude weights inevitably lead to only small changes in the calculated probability of disease. The effect can be very much greater for particular diagnostic problems, and if there is no adjustment completely misleading probabilities can be produced. Standard errors can also be calculated for both crude and adjusted weightings[21] and are shown for the adjusted weights in table 2.

An inspection of the crude weights given in table 2 also allows us to compare the symptoms. For example, the range of crude weights for sex is from -6 to $+5$, a range of 11. On the other hand, the range of weights for age, split in the way that it has been done, is from -10 to $+18$, a range of 28. The bigger the range of an indicant, the greater its potential value as a diagnostic item. The symptom conveying the least amount of evidence is the one derived by asking about the effect of food. The range there is only 8, considerably less than for the other symptoms shown.

Further analysis along these lines allows us to identify the most important symptoms for particular clinical problems, the selection of symptoms being something we should consider when teaching students. Many years ago Fletcher asked us to stop teaching and using unreliable signs, his advice coming from a rigorous assessment of variation among observers.[22] Perhaps others should now be left out— namely, those that convey little information when assessed in the way suggested above.

You might, however, see the limitations in regarding the importance of symptoms simply in terms of the range of weights that they provide. Clearly, it is possible to have a very powerful symptom that is so rarely present that it would not normally be ascertained in a routine clinical consultation. An example is given by Wilfrid Card, who once had a patient with steatorrhoea who presented because the patient had had to call the plumber to unblock the drain (as a result of the massive steatorrhoea). Clearly, if a patient gives this "symptom"—calling the plumber—then steatorrhoea is highly likely. Nobody, however, would consider it reasonable to ask patients in a general gastrointestinal clinic a direct question about whether they have had to call the plumber to unblock their lavatories.

What has been provided above are the weights to be applied to the relevant responses to a particular question.

Which is the best question?

The final step is then to consider the relative value of asking each question with respect to discovering whether a patient has the disease of interest. This is clearly related to two things—firstly, the weights of the various responses to that question as derived above, and, secondly, some measure of how common that symptom is in the disease of interest. (This gets round the problem posed by Card's symptom.) It is a slightly more complex subject than the derivation of crude weights, and you may wish to skip the next two paragraphs.

Calculating the relative value of asking each question is in fact a calculation of "the *expected* weight of evidence" from that question. This gives a single value for each question[23] and can be expressed by multiplying the probability that a particular response to a question will occur by the corresponding weight and adding in the same for each of the other possible responses to the same question. For example, the symptom of daily pain occurs in 21/235 cases of duodenal ulcer (table II). From adjusted weights (table II) the expected weight of evidence:

$$
\begin{aligned}
&= \left(\frac{21}{235} \times -11\right) + \left(\frac{214}{235} \times 2\right) \\
&= -0{\cdot}98 + 1{\cdot}82 \\
&= 0{\cdot}84 \text{ (always a positive value).}
\end{aligned}
$$

The sex of the patient gives a value of $0{\cdot}1$, and for the patient's age the expected weight of evidence is $4{\cdot}0$, much greater in fact than the other symptoms in the table. As it happens, age is a more useful piece of information to ask about than the patient's sex—which is obvious anyway.

In principle therefore the questions with the highest expected weight of evidence are clearly those that should be taught to medical students in the hope that they might be able to remember more easily those that are discriminating. Using these as signposts would help to guide them through the uncertainty that besets us all at some time or another when faced with a plethora of information, most of which has somehow to be discarded. These are the searchlights alluded to earlier,[1] which, if taught to students, can help us all.

Conclusion

It is probably unwise to speculate too much about future developments. Provided that the use of such systems is seen as a diagnostic aid, not a decision maker, and as a screening test or guide, not an automatic initiator of treatment or of further investigation, then these ideas will probably find a place in providing more efficient medical care for certain problems.

I acknowledge the financial support of the Scottish Home and Health Department and more recently of Smith, Kline and French. I am deeply indebted to my colleagues G P Crean, R J Holden, and D J Spiegelhalter for their contributions but most of all to the late W I Card, who pioneered the work described here.

1 Macartney F. Diagnostic logic. Br Med J 1987;295:1325-31.
2 Anonymous. Database on dyspepsia. [Editorial.] Br Med J 1978;i:1163-4.
3 de Dombal FT, Leaper DJ, Staniland JR, et al. Computer aided diagnosis of acute abdominal pain. Br Med J 1972;ii:9-13.
4 Adams ID, Chan M, Clifford PC, et al. Computer diagnosis of acute abdominal pain: a multicentre study. Br Med J 1986;293:800-4.
5 Lucas RW, Card WI, Knill-Jones RP, et al. Computer interrogation of patients. Br Med J 1976;ii:623-5.
6 Card WI, Lucas RW. Computer interrogation in medical practice. International Journal of Man-Machine Studies 1981;14:49-57.
7 Spiegelhalter DJ. Evaluation of clinical decision-aids, with an application to a system for dyspepsia. Stat Med 1983;2:207-15.
8 Knill-Jones RP, Dunwoodie WM, Crean GP. A computer assisted diagnostic decision system for dyspepsia. In: Sheldon M, Brooke J, Rector A, eds. Decision-making in general practice. London: Macmillan, 1985.
9 Spiegelhalter DJ. Statistical aids in clinical decision-making. The Statistician 1982;31:19-36.
10 Spiegelhalter DJ, Knill-Jones RP. Statistical and knowledge-based approaches to clinical decision-support systems with an application in gastroenterology. Journal of the Royal Statistical Society (Series A) 1984;147:35-77.
11 Brittain E. Probability of developing coronary heart disease. Stanford: Division of biostatistics, Stanford University, 1979. (Technical report No 54.)
12 Knill-Jones RP. A formal approach to symptoms in dyspepsia. Clin Gastroenterol 1985;14:517-9.
13 de Dombal FT. Analysis of symptoms in the acute abdomen. Clin Gastroenterol 1985;14:531-43.
14 Crean GP. Towards a positive diagnosis of irritable bowel syndrome. In: Read N, ed. Irritable bowel syndrome. New York: Grune and Stratton, 1985.
15 Card WI, Lucas RW, Spiegelhalter DJ. The logical description of a disease class as a Boolean function with special reference to the irritable bowel syndrome. Clin Sci 1984;66:307-15.
16 Knill-Jones RP, Maxwell JD, Thompson RPH, Williams R. Evaluation of a Bayesian model in the diagnosis of jaundice. Gut 1970;11:1062.
17 Knill-Jones RP, Stern RB, Girmes DH, et al. Use of sequential Bayesian model in diagnosis of jaundice by computer. Br Med J 1973;i:530-3.
18 Jennett B, Teasdale G, Braakman R, et al. Predicting outcome in individual patients after severe head injury. Lancet 1976;i:1031-4.
19 Matzen P, Malchow-Miller A, Hilden J, et al. Differential diagnosis of jaundice: a pocket diagnostic chart. Liver 1984;4:360-71.
20 Theodossi A, Knill-Jones RP, Skene A, et al. Inter-observer variation of symptoms and signs in jaundice. Liver 1981;1:21-32.
21 Spiegelhalter DJ. Statistical methodology for evaluating gastrointestinal symptoms. Clin Gastroenterol 1985;14:489-515.

22 Fletcher CM. The problem of observer variation in medical diagnosis with special reference to chest diseases. *Methods Inf Med* 1965;**3**:98-103.
23 Knill-Jones RP. A computer assisted diagnostic decision system for dyspepsia (GLADYS). *Lecture Notes in Medical Informatics* 1986;**28**:215-26.

Logic in medicine:
an economic perspective

ALAN MAYNARD

The Concise Oxford Dictionary defines logic as the science of thinking or a chain of reasoning or thought defensible on the grounds of consistency. Economics, at its best, is a logical way of analysing the costs and benefits of alternative ways of achieving competing objectives: it is the science of deciding how to allocate scarce means among competing ends.

Thomas Carlyle argued that economics was not a "gay science" but "the dismal science." Carlyle reached this conclusion because the basic assumptions of economics are scarcity and the ubiquitous necessity to make choices. In health care these factors require the allocators of resources to decide who will die and who will live in what degree of pain and discomfort.

Background

Expenditure on health care: international comparisons

During the past 40 years expenditure on health care in all Western countries has expanded rapidly, and in all cases the role of the state in financing and providing health care has increased so that even in the "capitalist" United States over 40 cents of each dollar spent on health care is provided by the government.

Comparative data on international expenditure on health care is notoriously complex because of differing definitions of health care and fluctuating exchange rates. Table 1 and the figure give a general picture of comparative expenditure in 1982.[2] In that year the amount

73

Table 1—Health care expenditure in selected Western countries[2]

	Expenditure per person in 1982 ($)*	Percentage of gross domestic product spent on health care in 1982	Elasticity of health care expenditure†
Australia	828	7·6	1·0
Belgium	534	6·2	2·3
Canada	989	8·2	1·6
Denmark	746	6·8	1·8
France	931	9·3	2·6
Germany	874	8·2	0·8
Ireland	436	8·2	1·0
Italy	441	7·2	0·8
Japan	602	6·6	1·4
New Zealand	440	5·7	
The Netherlands	836	8·7	0·7
United Kingdom	508	5·9	1·2
United States	1388	10·6	1·4
Sweden	1168	9·7	3·9
Switzerland	1158	7·8	

*Measured at current rates of exchange.
†Change in health care expenditure associated with a 1% growth in gross domestic product at constant prices during 1975-82.

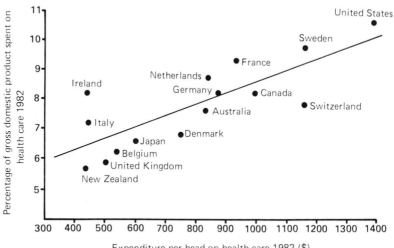

Comparative health care expenditure in selected Western countries, 1982. This graph shows that in a wide range of world economies a rich country (as judged by its gross domestic product in 1982 ($) at current rates of exchange) spends not only more on health care in absolute terms but also a higher *proportion* of its gross domestic product on health care: $r = 0.80$ ($p < 0.001$).

A similar graph exists for 1971.[19]

spent per person on health care in the United Kingdom was $508. This amount was similar to that in Belgium but only 54% of the amount spent per person in France, 58% of that in Germany, and 36% of that in the United States.

The proportion of gross domestic product spent on health care is less than 6% in the United Kingdom, over 8% in Germany, over 9% in France, and over 10% in the United States. These countries are spending high proportions of very much higher gross domestic products on health care, and this is the result of countries tending, as they get richer, to spend more on health care. The final column of table I shows that in most countries (even relatively poor ones like the United Kingdom) if the gross domestic product grows by 1% expenditure on health care (at least in 1975-82) grows by more than 1%.

One conclusion that can be derived from these data is that expenditure on health care is low because the United Kingdom is relatively poor and the rate of economic growth in the United Kingdom has been slow. Only if the growth rate in the United Kingdom becomes faster and its expenditure on health care mirrors international patterns will expenditure rise to the level of affluent states like France and Germany.

Expenditure on health care: domestic trends

The comparatively low expenditure on health care in the United Kingdom has grown unevenly in recent years. Table 2 shows the pattern of expenditure on health care since the 1983 election[3]: all the data have been adjusted to take account of inflation and pay increases. Expenditure on hospital care has been virtually static: level in 1983-4, it marginally declined in 1984-5 and grew by less than 0·5% in 1985-6.

Table 2—Recent expenditure changes (percentages) in NHS[3] (all data adjusted for change in prices and pay rates)

	Hospital and community health service	Family practitioner services	Total NHS	Local authority social services
1983-4	0·0	2·0	0·9	3·3
1984-5	0·1	2·8	1·4	1·5
1985-6	0·4	0·2	0·6	2·1

The government argues that an additional 1·5% a year of "growth" money has been generated by "efficiency savings"—that is, the recycling of funds from unproductive activities to more productive activities.

Expenditure on primary care in the National Health Service (NHS) is not cash limited but is open ended—that is, it depends on the number and behaviour of general practitioners and other contractors. The data in table 2 show that, except in 1985-6, real expenditure on primary care increased by over 2% each year in 1983-5. With the stock of general practitioners continuing to rise at about 1·8% a year this trend is likely to continue and cause anxiety to the controllers of public expenditure in Her Majesty's Treasury.

The cash limited budgets of local authority social services departments have grown unevenly since 1983. The growth in the real outlays of local authority social services (adjusting for inflation and pay changes) has never been less than 1·5%.

The increases in NHS (HCHS plus FPS) expenditure (hospital and community services and primary care) since 1983 has been modest yet important, particularly if efficiency savings of 1·5% a year are added in. The growth has been concentrated in the NHS primary care sector and local authority social services, and this may be appropriate, given the emphasis of policy on the development of high cost community care for priority groups such as the elderly, the mentally handicapped, and the mentally ill. At present the aggregate yearly budgets of the health care systems of England, Wales, Scotland, and Northern Ireland are over £20 000 million.

This level of expenditure, however, is inevitably inadequate for meeting all the competing demands for health care. Furthermore, the gap between provision and potential demand may be widening as the development of scientific knowledge and other factors increase the demands on scarce resources.

Sources of increased demand

Some of the sources of increased demand for care and cure provided by the NHS are as follows.

Demographic change—The "greying" of the population will result in there being more elderly people in the population and perhaps considerably increased levels of dependency, particularly for those aged 75 years and over. The estimated growth in hospital funding required to meet this demographic effect peaks in 1985-7 and requires at least a 1% real increase in funding, given the current patterns of expenditure. The pressure on expenditure from increased numbers of the elderly will fall for the next decade but will usually require 0·5% yearly increases in funding. With greater levels of dependency even this amount of funding may be inadequate.

Technological change—The effects of technological change on spending in the NHS, like the effects of elderly dependency, have been poorly researched. The Department of Health and Social Security asserts that the NHS requires a 0·5% increase in funding each year to finance technological advances. The scientific basis of this advocacy, however, which is apparently accepted by the Treasury, is absent: it is a crude estimate.

Community care—Since the 1970s successive governments have pursued a policy of developing community care for the elderly, the mentally ill, and the mentally handicapped. Initially it was thought that this policy would reduce costs, but now it is clear that it is very much more expensive—for example, the average annual cost of institutional care for a mentally ill person is £12 000, but care in the community costs £16 000-£20 000. These higher costs are partly the result of providing care in small community units, where there are fewer economies of scale. Community care may also be of higher quality, though this aspect of provision has not been evaluated. The escalating cost of these programmes will drain resources from the sector dealing with acute illnesses, and it is pressures such as these that may lead to the "reinvention" of institutional care, though I hope this will not lead to the reinvention of the comparative neglect that such a policy seems to have produced in the recent past.

Acquired immune deficiency syndrome—The average cost of treating a patient who has the acquired immune deficiency syndrome (AIDS) once he enters the health care system is about £20 000. The average length of life is about 400 days, and the number of cases is rising rapidly. This epidemic will require considerable new resources if existing services are not to be rationed even more carefully.

Screening for breast cancer and cervical cytology screening—The evidence from Scandinavia indicates that breast screening for post-menopausal women will save lives. The Forrest committee has recommended introducing a selective breast screening programme. Evidence from research also shows that cervical cancer is a much

77

greater problem than was thought five years ago. Consequently, there is a need not only to improve the levels of screening of women aged over 35 (particularly those in poorer socioeconomic groups) but also to extend screening to all women aged 20 and over. The effects on resources of introducing breast cancer screening and extending cytology screening are considerable.

Reforms in nurse training—The nursing profession is facing two problems. Firstly, it wishes to upgrade its training standards, making more nurses take degree courses. Secondly, owing to demographic trends and existing entry requirements the number of young people entering the profession will fall by up to one quarter in the next five years. More resources are therefore required to fund degree training and make up for the loss of student nurses on the ward and to increase the supply of nurses and carers (for example, by paying higher wages) to remedy the ravages of demography.

Reducing inequalities in primary health care and local authority social services—Considerable inequalities exist in the geographical distribution of the provision of local authority social services and primary care. The Social Services Select Committee examined the distribution of local authority social services provision and argued that these inequalities should be removed by the government.[4] Birch and Maynard have shown that substantial inequalities exist in the primary care provided in England and that a policy of equality would shift resources and general practitioners from the south to the north.[5] The paradox is that policies to equalise the distribution of health care resources (for example, the Resource Allocation Working Party in England and Scottish Health Authorities Revenue Equalisation in Scotland) have been directed at hospital resources alone. The inequalities in the provision of social services and primary care are substantial, and any attempt to reduce them may affect resources considerably.

Preventing illness and promoting health—Another area generating demand for new resources is health education and promotion. The problem of AIDS has led to the creation (from April 1987) of a new health authority which, in England, has taken over the role of the former Health Education Council and is concerned with preventing the spread of AIDS. At present about 100 000 people die prematurely because of their smoking habits,[6] maybe as many as 40 000 people die prematurely because of their drinking (alcohol) habits,[7] but fewer than 150 die prematurely as a result of their use of illicit drugs. The emphasis of existing policies on prevention seems to be unbalanced, but obviously the costs to governments of challenging powerful corporate interests are not inconsiderable in terms of financial support and votes. The subjects of illness prevention and health promotion are complex, but there are important opportunities to purchase considerable improvements in the length and quality of life at low cost, as is seen below (see table 5).

There are, then, demands from many groups for additional funding. Such additional funding would enable the NHS to provide health care treatments and programmes that could generate appreciable improvements in the health of the population. These programmes and other demands articulated throughout the Service cannot, however, be financed. The resources are not available to meet all the demands made by health care.

The nature of economic logic

Scarcity

It is the ubiquitous nature of scarcity that is the starting point of economic analysis. Of course NHS funds could be augmented by switching defence funds to health care or switching private consumption on videos, junk food, and foreign holidays via taxation to provision for the NHS. Such switches, even if socially acceptable, would not abolish scarcity but merely alter its nature. Even the Americans, who are spending 2·7 times as much per person on health, ration care, particularly for those whose ability to pay for it is limited.

Criteria for choice

Once scarcity is accepted the consequence is that there will always be medical interventions that, although productive in the sense that they enhance the quality and quantity of life, cannot be funded. Decisions have to be made about which types of health care will be provided. The debate must then be about the principles or criteria that will be used to choose which patients will get what care when.

Opportunity costs

Any choice results in an opportunity cost equal to the value of the alternative that is foregone. The opportunity cost of the Trident programme is fewer resources available for the NHS, videos, and roads. More health care for the priority groups means that fewer resources are available for patients who have acute illnesses. More diagnostic provision—for instance, the acquisition of a magnetic resonance imaging scanner—leaves less money available to fund other parts of the hospital system. There is no such thing as a free lunch: every choice results in an opportunity cost. In the case of the "free" lunch the opportunity cost is your time.

Economic efficiency

Choices have to be informed by information about the costs and benefits of each alternative. Such information enables the decision maker to identify the most efficient option. The pursuit of efficient practices is not merely about reducing costs; if it were, the most "efficient" procedure would be to do nothing, as that pushes costs to zero. Efficiency is defined as the minimum cost of producing a given outcome or the maximisation of outcomes from a given budget. Thus the achievement of economic efficiency requires the minimisation of costs and the maximisation of outcomes (or benefits).

Inefficiency is unethical

The consequence of scarcity is that choices have to be made, and efficient choices seem to be the most desirable: they maximise benefits (improvements in health) from a given budget. If doctors do not evaluate their practices and strive for this goal their practices may be inefficient. Inefficiency means that costs are not minimised and benefits are not maximised: in other words, there is waste of scarce resources. Waste, or inefficiency, means that potential patients (in the queue for care) are deprived of health care from which they could benefit. Inefficiency in one hospital department may mean that resources are not available for orthopaedics and that patients are left in avoidable disability and distress.

Inefficiency is unethical. If patients are not to be deprived of care from which they could benefit doctors must make evaluation and efficiency the priorities that dominate their practices.

Identifying efficiency: theory and the margin

When making decisions on allocation we need information about costs and benefits (outcomes). Before considering how to identify and measure these variables, however, it is necessary to decide what data are actually needed for decision making.

The managers, administrators, and clinicians of a health care system typically generate data in terms of totals and averages (arithmetic means). The first rule for achieving economic efficiency with such data is:

(1) (a) if total costs exceed total benefits do not invest in the procedure;

(b) if total benefits exceed total costs do invest in the procedure.

This does not, however, tell us what amount to invest if rule 1(b) is met. The advice of the economist is that the decision on the level of investment should be decided by using data about the margin. The margin is the increment added to either costs or outcomes by a small (one unit) change in the level of activity. Thus the decision maker needs data on the marginal cost of producing one more (or one fewer) hernia repair and the marginal benefit to the state of health of one more or one fewer of such a procedure. From these data the second rule may be derived to decide the efficient level of investment in an activity:

(2) (a) if marginal cost exceeds marginal benefit reduce investment;

(b) if marginal benefit exceeds marginal cost increase investment;

(c) when marginal cost equals marginal benefit stop investing and maintain that efficient level of output.

The logic of these rules is quite simple. Rule 2 (a) indicates that if, as a result of increasing activity by one unit (the margin), the value of opportunity costs (foregone alternatives) exceeds the benefits of the procedure investment could be made more productively elsewhere and the level of activity should be reduced. On the other hand, if the benefits (in terms of the incremental effects on the state of health) exceed the costs of one more operation investment in that procedure should increase. The efficient level of activity is where costs and benefits are equal at the margin.

Identifying efficiency: using the margin in decision making

Are such theoretical rules of any use in determining the level and nature of the allocation of resources in the NHS, or is the logic of theory useless in practice? There are inevitably problems in applying such rules, but their power and usefulness in informing decision making can be shown by a simple example.

In the late 1960s data from trials in the United States identified the cost and outcome (in terms of identifying cancers) of the use of the guaiac stool test as a screening device to identify cancer of the colon. Table 3 shows these data.[8] The policy debate surrounding these data was what level of guaiac testing to adopt as efficient practice. Carrying out more tests increased costs but also reduced false negative results in cancer detection. Table 3 shows that the average cost per cancer detected rose from $1175 to $2451, and the opinion was that doing six stool guaiac tests was "good practice."

Simple manipulation of these data using the concept of the margin shows nicely how useful economic logic can be. In table 4 the second column shows the increase in the number of cancers found from each additional (marginal) test. The next column shows how costs increased with marginal increases in testing. The final column shows that the cost of identifying a marginal (one more) case of cancer rose from $1175 with one test to $47m with six tests.

Early intervention in this cancer saves lives, but is it worth

Table 3—Test results and costs of stool guaiac tests[8]

No of tests	No of cancers found	No of cancers missed (false negatives)	Total cost of diagnosis ($)	Average cost per cancer ($)
1	65·946	5·99500	77511	1175
2	71·442	0·49960	107690	1507
3	71·900	0·04160	130199	1811
4	71·938	0·00350	148116	2059
5	71·941	0·00030	163141	2268
6	71·942	0·00003	176331	2451

Table 4—Marginal results and costs for subsequent stool guaiac tests[8]

No of tests	Increase in No of cancers found	Increase in total costs ($)	Marginal cost per cancer found ($)
1	65·94600	77 511	1 175
2	5·49600	30 179	5 491
3	0·45800	22 509	49 146
4	0·03800	17 917	471 500
5	0·00372	15 025	4 038 978
6	0·00028	13 190	47 107 143

spending $47m to save one more life? All these data are in 1968 prices, and with or without adjustment for inflation the cost of this screening activity when it includes six tests seems to be high. Without using the concept of the margin, however, this cost is not identified, and inefficient decisions may be made.

Identifying efficiency: measuring costs and benefits

In this example the measurement of cost refers only to the guaiac procedure, and the measurement of outcome is the number of cancers identified. Both of these measures, though useful, are crude.

In evaluating a procedure the full costs have to be identified. What is the cost of treating a case of head and neck cancer? To cost just the hospital surgery is incomplete. The costs of this need to be added to the costs of hospital diagnosis, referral costs in primary care and post-operative care, and the non-NHS costs—that is, the costs associated with local authority social services, the care provided by voluntary agencies (for example, hospices), and the costs to the patient and the household in which he normally lives. The objective of the costing is to identify the effect on resources of the relevant episode of illness.

The problems associated with costing a procedure, though not inconsiderable, are fewer than those arising from evaluating the outcome. The guaiac case takes as a measure of benefit the identification of a case of cancer of the colon. Indeed, it is commonplace throughout medical evaluation to use intermediate outcome measures and indicators such as survival. The outcome of a health care intervention, however, is not merely survival but the quality of that survival: General Franco, the Spanish dictator, was kept alive by technology for the last 80 days of his life, the quality of which, as he was mostly unconscious, was very low.

In the late 1970s the United States Office of Technology Assessment introduced the concept of the QALY—that is, the quality adjusted life year.[9] For example, one year of full quality life would be free from disability and distress. This was a measure of outcome that combined measuring the additional life years associated with a procedure with their quality. The measurement of the quality of life is crude and may be as inaccurate as the measurement of the quantity of life (survival). The virtue of such measures, however, is that they are explicit, and consequently the debate about the allocation of resources is about objective problems such as the measurement of quality of life and cost rather than subjective and about the political power of doctors competing for resources.

The methods used to estimate the cost of quality adjusted life years are detailed elsewhere.[10 11] Tables 5 and 4 set out some results. The data in table 5 are the result of work by Williams,[10 12] who has applied the pioneering work of Rosser and Kind[13] to a variety of treatments in

Table 5—Data on cost per quality adjusted life year (QALY) United Kingdom, 1983-4[10 12]

	Cost per QALY (£)
Hip replacement	750
Pacemaker implantation for arterioventricular heart block	700
Valve replacement for aortic stenosis	900
Coronary artery bypass grafts for:	
Severe angina with left main vessel disease	1 040
Severe angina with three vessel disease	1 270
Moderate angina with left main vessel disease	1 330
Severe angina with two vessel disease	2 280
Moderate angina with three vessel disease	2 400
Mild angina with left main vessel disease	2 520
Action by general practitioner:	
Advice to stop smoking	167
Control of hypertension	1 700
Control of total serum cholesterol	1 700
Kidney transplant	3 200
Heart transplant	5 000
Hospital haemodialysis	14 000

Table 6—Estimates of cost per quality adjusted life year (QALY) North America, 1983[14]

	Cost per QALY ($)
Coronary artery bypass graft for left main coronary artery disease	4 200
Neonatal intensive care (1000-1499 g)	4 500
Thyroxine (thyroid screening)	6 300
Treatment for severe hypertension in men aged >40 years (diastolic pressure 105 mm Hg)	19 100
Treatment for mild hypertension (94-105 mm Hg)	19 100
Oestrogen treatment for postmenopausal symptoms in women without previous hysterectomy	27 000
Neonatal intensive care (500-999 g)	31 800
Coronary artery bypass graft for single vessel disease, moderately severe	36 300
School tuberculin testing programme	43 700
Continuous ambulatory peritoneal dialysis	47 100
Hospital dialysis	54 000

the United Kingdom. Table 6 summarises data from North America and draws on the work of Torrance at McMaster University.[14]

These results are inevitably controversial. For instance, the North American data indicate that intensive neonatal care for low birth-weight children (500-999 g) is an expensive way to produce a QALY, though it is less expensive than hospital dialysis and continuous ambulatory peritoneal dialysis treatment for patients who have end stage renal failure.

From Williams's estimates some very clear priorities are established for the allocation of (especially marginal) NHS resources. If a district had £1m growth money and only the options listed in table 5 to spend this money on, its managers would recognise that it could produce 5988 QALYs from advice by general practitioners to stop smoking, 1333 QALYs from hip replacements, and 71 QALYs from hospital dialysis. Clearly, a health authority wishing to maximise QALYs (improvements in health) would invest its £1m in advice by general practitioners to stop smoking.

Some would reject such measures as generating unsatisfactory criteria to determine the allocation of resources.[15] But are cost-QALY criteria any more unsatisfactory than existing measures, which are ad hoc, incoherent, and inconsistent? Some health authorities think not and are using this approach to help in decisions about allocating resources.[11]

The implications of economics for the NHS

Economic analysis offers an explicit framework for appraising decisions about the use of scarce resources. It obliges decision makers to define objectives, assumed to be efficiency or the maximisation of improvements in health (QALYs), from a finite £20 billion NHS budget but to incorporate distributional (equity) issues as desired.[5] Furthermore, it requires careful evaluation of the full (opportunity) costs of competing treatments and the identification and measurement (even if crudely) of outcomes (QALYs).

Identifying efficient practices, however, does not mean that the behaviour of doctors will be efficient: you can lead a horse to water but you cannot make it drink. To ensure that the behaviour of the hospital clinician and general practitioner is consistent with the findings of evaluative research practitioners may have to be "persuaded" with cash incentives and non-financial rules. For instance, general practitioners could be persuaded to take a greater interest in the higher incidence of cervical cancer in poor women if they were paid not just for each cervical cytology test but for identifying positive results. Non-financial regulations could include setting performance norms, rigorous peer review, and short term renewable contracts of employment for doctors.

It is inevitable that the NHS employment market will become more uncertain because policy makers require greater responsiveness from providers and greater flexibility in the provision of services. The role of the profession and its practitioners will be challenged, and the role of the consumer will be increasingly to question decisions and demand the evaluative (cost-QALY) information on which they are based. Adam Smith posed a dilemma nicely when he wrote in 1776:

The pretence that corporations are necessary for the better government of the trade is without foundation. The real and effectual discipline which is exercised over the workman, is not that of his corporation, but that of his customers. It is the fear of losing their employment which restrains his frauds and corrects his negligence.

In addition to the increased pressure for evaluating treatments and incentives the application of economics to health care will create the need for better medical education. At present most medical schools offer little in the way of systematic teaching of economics to young doctors.[16] Similarly, there is all too little systematic teaching of economics at postgraduate level and during careers. Knowledge of economics is required for two reasons: firstly, to "immunise" doctors against the results of bad economic analysis, and, secondly, to enable doctors to participate in comprehensive, collaborative trials of the costs and benefits of treatments and programmes.

The immediate response to such a proposal is that the medical school curriculum is already full, and so it is. But what is the opportunity cost of not teaching economics, and what is the value at the margin of teaching economics vis à vis other inputs in medical education? For most doctors some economic knowledge may be of more use during their lifetime than esoteric aspects of surgery and medicine that become redundant after successfully completing examinations.

Economic analysis, like medicine, is scientific, but, like medicine, the margins of error may be considerable (for example, estimates of premature mortality related to alcohol range from an estimate derived from official sources of fewer than 8000[17] to 25 000[18] to 40 000[7] a year). Like doctors, economists are working to reduce the margins of error in an attempt to improve the allocation of scarce resources among competing demanders. A major virtue of economic analysis is that it is an explicit framework that is logical—that is, defensible on the grounds of consistency. Its social perspective inevitably challenges the individual perspective of the doctor, but such challenges are not a threat to the medical profession; rather, they are an incentive to improve understanding and, by careful evaluation, improve the quality and quantity of care available for patients.

1 Carlyle T. The Nigger Question. *Frazers Magazine* 1849;**40**:670-9. Reprinted in: August ER, ed. *Carlyle The Nigger Question, Still The Negro Question.* New York: Appleton Century Crofts, 1971.
2 Organisation for Economic Cooperation and Development. *Measuring health care: expenditure, costs and performance.* Paris: OECD, 1985. (Social Policy Studies No 2.)
3 Department of Health and Social Security. Evidence to the House of Commons Select Committee on the Social Services. London: HMSO 1986. (House of Commons Paper 387 1985-6 Session.)
4 Select Committee on Social Services. *Public expenditure.* London: HMSO, 1986.
5 Birch S, Maynard A. *The RAWP review: RAWPing the UK and RAWPing primary care.* York: Centre for Health Economics, University of York, 1986. (Discussion Paper No 19.)
6 Royal College of Physicians. *Health or smoking?* London: Pitman, 1983.
7 Royal College of General Practitioners. *Alcohol: a balanced view.* London: RCGP, 1986.
8 Newhauser O, Lewicki M. National health insurance and the sixth stool guaiac. *Policy Analysis* 1976;**24**:175-96.
9 Office of Technology Assessment. *A review of selected federal vaccine and immunization policies.* Washington, DC: United States Congress, 1979.
10 Williams A. Economics of coronary artery bypass grafting. *Br Med J* 1985;**291**:326-9.
11 Gudex C. *QALYs and their use by the health service.* York: Centre for Health Economics, University of York. 1986 (Discussion Paper No 20.)
12 Williams A. Screening for risk of coronary heart disease: is it a wise use of resources? In: Oliver M, Ashley-Miller M, Wood D, eds. *Screening for risk of coronary heart disease.* London: Wiley, 1986.
13 Rosser RM, Kind P. A scale of valuation of states of illness: is there a social consensus? *Int J Epidemiol,* 1978;**7**:347-57.

14 Torrance GW. Measurement of health state utilities for economic appraisal: a review. *Journal of Health Economics* 1986;5:1-30.
15 O'Donnell M. *Doctor, doctor: an insider's view of games people play.* London: Victor Gollancz, 1986.
16 Spoor C, Mooney G, Maynard A. Teaching health economics. *Br Med J* 1986;**292**:785.
17 McDonnell R, Maynard A. Estimation of life years lost. *Alcohol and Alcoholism* 1985;**20**:435-43.
18 Royal College of Psychiatrists. *Alcohol: our favourite drug.* London: RCP, 1986.
19 Golding AMB. Decision making in the NHS. *Br Med J* 1984;**288**:203-7.

Fundamental ethical principles in health care

IAN E THOMPSON

The title of this paper seems to beg at least two questions.

(1) Is there sufficient common ground among the medical, nursing, paramedical, chaplaincy, and social work professions to justify looking for ethical principles common to "health care"?

(2) Do we really have sufficient logical grounds, or consensus among health workers and the public, to speak of "fundamental ethical principles in health care"?

Both questions will be examined in an attempt to clarify which requirements of morality are logically primary, or fundamental, to the ethics of health care. In colloquial usage the term "principle" is used very loosely to cover moral rules or demands that may be either logically fundamental or derived. Thus the seemingly repetitive phrase "fundamental principles" is used to clarify the distinction between the two.

Cultural and historical relativities in professional ethics

At first sight the ethical codes evolved in medicine, particularly in the Hippocratic tradition, and similar codes evolved more recently by nurses and the paramedical professions seem to be as much concerned with underpinning the identity and defending the interests of the relevant professional groups as with patients' or clients' rights.[1-8] If we focus attention on the attempts made in each to demarcate roles and responsibilities and to defend professional territory then it is difficult to see how it would be possible to arrive at any common principles of ethics of health care. We seem to be confronted with a series of independent "language games" of ethical discourse with constitutive principles and rules peculiar to each profession and the role responsibilities of each.

A functional or sociological analysis of the content of such codes would tend to emphasise the relativity of the "principles" invoked by each profession and would tend to explain the differences and common features among them in terms of the relative positions of the different professional groups in the power structure of the health services in any given society. Further, a historical analysis of the emergence of nursing, social work, and the paramedical professions would tend to highlight how, in the struggle to achieve an independent professional identity, these professions have had to contend with the dominant medical profession to negotiate and achieve a workable division of labour in each different system of health care.[9]

All this would tend to emphasise the relativity, historical contingency, and culturally specific character of any principles embodied in the different codes of health professionals.

The Hippocratic "tradition"

Similarly, an examination of the historical tradition of medical ethics, for example, would bring to light how confused and discontinuous it has been. Doctors like to boast of the continuity of the tradition of medical ethics stretching back over more than 2000 years to Hippocrates (about 420 BC). Closer examination, however, shows that the Hippocratic oath* was peculiar to only one of several schools of medicine in antiquity. The Hippocratic tradition was virtually forgotten until reintroduced to Europe by the Arabs in the eleventh century. With the establishment of universities and schools of medicine in mediaeval Europe Roger II of Sicily in 1140 and Frederick II of Germany attempted to control medical practice, and at the time certain guilds of doctors adopted the Hippocratic oath as a basis for membership of the profession. At about the same time the church gave general endorsement to the oath, particularly because of its proscriptions of abortion and euthanasia.

The oath was never subscribed to universally, and after the Reformation and the fragmentation of Europe into nation states during the sixteenth and seventeenth centuries the Hippocratic tradition was more honoured in the breach than the observance. Only in the nineteenth century, with the development of modern scientific

*See page 95.

medicine and the struggle among doctors, surgeons, and apothecaries for professional dominance, did the oath re-emerge as the basis of the doctors' code of practice. It was a self conscious attempt at the time to invest medicine with a respectable image based in a scientific and ethical tradition going back to the Greeks.[10][11] Although based ostensibly on the Hippocratic oath, the Declaration of Geneva (1948) of the newly formed World Medical Association speaks only of respect for human life from the time of conception and avoids commitment on the controversial issues of abortion, suicide, and euthanasia.[12] So much for the sacred tradition.

Between the fundamentalists of the (recent) Hippocratic tradition and the liberals, such as the authors of the Declaration of Geneva and others who have been willing further to dilute or relativise the requirements of the original oath, there have been tensions and disagreements as strong as those between fundamentalists and liberals in religion. Further complicating the picture is the explicit teaching on medical ethics by the Catholic church and orthodox Judaism. Protestant contributions to the debate have been various but without a specific body of principles being enunciated—and this is not to mention evolved and evolving traditions within Islamic, Chinese, and traditional medicine in other cultures.

The picture seems to be one of such moral and cultural diversity that it may seem to be inherently implausible to suggest that there might be underlying ethical principles common to health care as such.

Evidence of emerging consensus on principles

Several developments in the past 50 years have, however, pointed to the emergence of a consensus about values and principles in health care that cuts across sectional, national, and cultural differences and even suggests broad agreement about fundamental ethical principles.

World Medical Association

The evidence that emerged in the Nuremberg war crimes tribunal of appalling atrocities committed by Nazi doctors in the pursuit of so called scientific research and their abuse of clinical responsibility in their cooperation in torture and forced "experiments" in genetic research provoked not only public outrage but a restatement in several declarations of the World Medical Association of ethical principles common to doctors everywhere.[12] The Nuremberg Code (1947) restated the principle of informed and voluntary consent to treatment; the principle that experiments should be conducted only if they were "such as to yield fruitful results for the good of society" and if these results were unobtainable by other means; and, further, requirements that experiments should be conducted according to strict scientific methods and by competently qualified persons.

The Declaration of Geneva (1948) paraphrased the Hippocratic oath in rather bland general terms but emphasised the principles of confidentiality; non-discrimination on grounds of race, religion, political affiliation, or social standing; and respect for human life from the time of conception. Other later declarations elaborated on these principles in relation to several specific problems and practical applications, without perhaps adding any new principles.

The Declaration of Helsinki (1964) further elaborated the criteria for scientifically and ethically sound medical research with human subjects, attempting to clarify the distinction between therapeutic and non-therapeutic clinical research. The Declaration of Sydney (1968) attempted a statement on the definition of death (with reference to the recent developments of artificial life support systems and organ transplantation). The Declaration of Oslo (1970) attempted to square the demand for therapeutic abortion with the Hippocratic tradition, and the Declarations of Tokyo (1975) and Hawaii (1977) represented statements proscribing the participation of doctors (or members of the World Medical Association) in torture or other cruel or degrading treatment or punishment of prisoners; and, seeking to limit the abuse of psychiatric treatment, to enforce ideological conformity.

These statements of principle by the World Medical Association are put forward without historical or philosophical justification as self evident truths. The fact that they have been given wide endorsement by the profession world wide (in theory if not always in practice) suggests several possibilities—namely, that they might be self evident truths or simply bland truisms to which assent can easily be given; or that the values of Western medicine are sufficiently globally disseminated that the profession *qua* profession acknowledges a similar value base to its practice wherever modern medicine is practised; or that these statements of principle represent the emergence of a genuine moral consensus that transcends cultural, religious, and national differences.

Emergence of other health care professions

In nursing, social work, and the paramedical professions there has been a similar process of formulating codes of practice and statements of fundamental values and ethical principles. It is beyond the scope of this paper to discuss these in detail, but it is perhaps interesting to note these developments at national and international level. Further, the World Health Organisation has recently played an important part in helping this process in medicine and nursing and encouraging other professions allied to medicine to address ethical issues in practice.[1-8] The International Council of Nurses formulated its *Code for Nurses* in 1953,[2] and subsequently national nursing bodies followed suit—for example, the American Nurses' Association (1968)[3] and the Royal College of Nursing (1979).[4] Clinical psychologists were led by the American Psychological Association (1977),[5] and other national bodies have followed with adaptations of their basic code. The British Association of Social Workers issued its *Code of Ethics for Social Workers* in 1975[6] and *Confidentiality in Social Work* in 1977.[7] The Central Council for Education and Training in Social Work also published *Values in Social Work* (1976).[8] The other professions allied to medicine—physiotherapy, speech therapy, occupational therapy, chiropody, dietetics, and health education—have each begun developing similar codes, the Society of Health Education Officers having issued a discussion document on ethics in health education in 1986.

It may be argued that this fashion for codes of ethics simply mimics medicine, not only in terms of seeking professional credibility and respectability by "professing" a code of ethics but also in broadly following the principles that belong to the analysis of the caring relationship and its obligations within medicine and the Hippocratic tradition. If this is so the emerging consensus on principles in health care may be apparent rather than real and based anyway on imitation and adaptation of medical codes rather than original differences or novel insights.

Against this it can be pointed out that in both nursing and social work the codes in question require a much more explicit recognition of patients' or clients' rights—for example, the right to know, the right to privacy, and the right to adequate care. Social workers and psychologists have probably explored much more fully the nature and implications of confidentiality, health educators the right to information and self help, and nurses in particular the health workers' role as an advocate of the rights of the vulnerable individual and the responsibility to work to restore autonomy to the patient who has lost it by virtue of injury, disease, or mental disorder.

Regulating biomedical research—the American experience

Public concern and media publicity about the use of prisoners as research subjects resulted in the setting up by the United States government of a National Commission for the Protection of Human Subjects of Biomedical and Behavioural Research. Faced with the apparent cultural diversity and relativity of principles professed in health care and the biomedical sciences, the commission had to formulate guidelines for the Department of Health, Education, and Welfare.

The Belmont report, which represents the collected research of the commission over several years, states an interesting consensus view that emerged over fundamental principles among members of the multiprofessional and interdisciplinary commission[13] (it represented a wide variety of health workers, lawyers, philosophers, theologians, and social scientists). They enunciated the principles of beneficence, justice, and respect for persons as fundamental to the ethics of health care and argued the case in convincing detail in several reports that other ethical principles could either be derived from or reduced to these.

Historical, cultural, and logical grounds for fundamental principles

Now the fact that one commission (and an American one at that) has argued that beneficence, justice, and respect for persons are basic or fundamental ethical principles does not prove anything in itself (leaving aside the volumes of research papers supporting the Belmont report). Such a consensus might reflect only a consensus among members of the commission or among Americans and not have universal application. If this view is defensible it must, firstly, be compatible with the historical evidence; secondly, make sense of cultural diversity and evident moral relativities; and, finally, be logically coherent.

In the remainder of this paper I shall consider each of these issues in turn and finally conclude with a brief discussion of some of the practical implications of the three basic principles.

Historical arguments—the Hippocratic tradition

When considering the historical evidence it may be instructive to begin with the Hippocratic oath itself.[14] There are various versions of the oath, but the following may be taken as representative:

I swear by Apollo the physician, by Aesculapius, Hygeia and Panacea, and I take to witness all the gods, all the goddesses, to keep according to my ability and my judgment the following Oath:

To consider dear to me as my parents him who taught me this art; to live in common with him and if necessary to share my goods with him; to look upon his children as my own brothers, to teach them this art if they so desire without fee or written promise; to impart to my sons and the sons of the master who taught me and the disciples who have enrolled themselves and have agreed to the rules of the profession, but to these alone, the precepts and the instruction. I will prescribe regimen for the good of my patients according to my ability and my judgment and never do harm to anyone. To please no one will I prescribe a deadly drug, nor give advice which may cause his death. Nor will I give a woman a pessary to procure abortion. But I will preserve the purity of my life and my art. I will not cut for stone, even for patients in whom the disease is manifest, I will leave this operation to be performed by practitioners (specialists in this art). In every house where I come I will enter only for the good of my patients, keeping myself far from all intentional ill-doing and all seduction, and especially from the pleasures of love with women or with men, be they free or slaves. All that may come to my knowledge in the exercise of my profession or outside of my profession or in daily commerce with men, which ought not to be spread abroad, I will keep secret and will never reveal. If I keep this oath faithfully, may I enjoy my life and practise my art, respected by all men and in all times; but if I swerve from it or violate it, may the reverse be my lot.

Firstly, it is interesting to note how the doctor hedges his bets by swearing in the names of the god of the physicians (Apollo), the god of the surgeons (Aesculapius), and the goddesses of prevention (Hygeia) and cure all (Panacea). The next part of the oath represents a classic statement of the case for a closed shop, based on medical protectionism and a monopoly in the control of medical knowledge and practical skills.

We see here at the very beginning a tension in medicine between the exoteric character of medicine as a self styled scientific discipline and the esoteric character of the profession as a semisecret masonic brotherhood based on charisma and magic. It is important to remember that the Hippocratic school was closed to all but those prepared to undergo the prescribed religious rituals and rites of initiation. Only then could access be gained to medical knowledge and training in the secret skills of the physician or surgeon. The amusement of modern medical students at the idea that their respect for their teachers should extend to a commitment to give them and their offspring financial support and free medical training springs from an awareness of this peculiar tension: on the one hand the secret, cultic, magic side of medicine as an art (the charism or placebo effect of the drug "doctor" still being the most potent instrument in the doctor's armamentarium[15]); and, on the other, the open, scientific, experimental side of medicine as a science (based on replicable experiments, controlled trials, and openly published and testable results).

The most specifically ethical prescriptions of the oath may readily be grouped under the three principles of beneficence, justice, and respect for persons.

The duty to do good and avoid doing harm (beneficence or nonmaleficence)—"I will prescribe regimen for the good of my patients according to my ability and judgment and never do harm to anyone."

"In every house where I come I will enter only for the good of my patients, keeping myself far from all intentional ill-doing. . . ."

Fairness to all or non-discrimination (justice)—The references are to the non-exploitation of the vulnerable, particularly women, children, and slaves (including any kind of sexual abuse). Further, the commitment not to pretend to skills the doctor lacks: "I will not cut for stone . . . but leave this operation to be performed by practitioners (specialists in this art)."

Respect for life and the dignity of patients (respect for persons)—"To please no one will I prescribe a deadly drug, nor give advice which may cause his death. Nor will I give a woman a pessary to procure abortion." (These are interpreted widely as proscriptions against euthanasia, assisted suicide, and abortion.)

"All that may come to my knowledge in the exercise of my profession . . . which ought not to be spread abroad, I will keep secret and never reveal." (This is recognition of the patient's right to privacy and the doctor's duty to maintain confidentiality.)

A detailed analysis of the extant declarations of the World Medical Association will show that the various principles enunciated can be derived from the three principles of beneficence, justice, and respect for persons or represent concrete applications of them. For example, the principle that subjects of biomedical research or recipients of medical treatment should give informed and voluntary consent is a corollary of the principle of respect for persons; the principle of non-discrimination on grounds of race, religion, and so on a corollary of the principle of justice; and the requirement that the doctor should accept full responsibility for treatments prescribed for incompetent patients or for any research subjects is a requirement of the principle of beneficence.

Gillon, in his otherwise excellent series on philosophical medical ethics, takes for granted the primacy of the three basic principles without showing whence they originate, how they are interrelated, or how other issues he discusses are related to these principles.[16-23] He seems to assume that it is intuitively self evident that these principles are fundamental to medical ethics. The interdependence of the principle of beneficence and non-maleficence ("primum non nocere") can be shown to be positive and negative formulations of the same principle. The requirement of truth telling or honesty is likewise derived from the principle of honour or respect for the patient as a person with a right to know. It is tempting, particularly within the fairly intact and conformist values of British medicine, to take for granted as self evident truths the principles on which our tradition is based and to use a kind of circular intuitionist argument to justify these principles as fundamental. Other kinds of demonstration are needed to justify the claim that beneficence, justice, and respect for persons are basic principles.

Cultural analysis—the evolution of principles

Cultural analysis can be offered to show the evolution of these three principles in ethical systems of widely different kinds. There was a time, earlier in this century, when arguments to the effect that all

97

ethical principles are relative and culturally specific were useful to challenge the cultural and moral imperialism of the West. Today it is more urgent not only to find common principles on which to found peace and disarmament and to ensure human survival on this planet but also to create international agencies. The formulation of, for example, the UN Declaration of Human Rights, the development of international law, and a revival of interest in the concepts of natural law bear testimony to a growing global consensus about fundamental human values and common ethical principles. Even moral philosophers (who perhaps have a vested interest in keeping a free market economy in moral systems going) are beginning to reflect a growing recognition that beneficence, justice, and respect for persons are in a sense basic to what ethics in general, and the ethics of health care in particular, is about.[24][25]

This is perhaps not surprising if we reflect both on the evolution of human beings within the structure of the family and tribal societies and on the broader history of our own Western culture. In all human societies people are born, grow to maturity, reproduce, become old, and die. These common features of human experience alone suggest that there are likely to be commonalities in the way that we perceive values or the conditions that make possible human flourishing. In family life and tribal society the quasiparental duty to care—for children, the weak, and the vulnerable—is taken for granted as being basic to social organisation and necessary for survival of the species. As children grow to maturity and seek recognition of their rights and a place for themselves in society so the demands of public justice (for liberty, equality, fraternity) begin to emerge. As people acquire more power and share in their society and are able to exercise more independent responsibility, and particularly as roles are reversed and the older generation become more dependent, the issue of respect for individual dignity and autonomy of people as people becomes an important issue in society.

In family and tribal life, religious orders, and hierarchical and monarchical societies the offer of a protective beneficence by the ruler of the community requires a matching duty of cooperative obedience in those subject to his or her rule. Here beneficence is the pre-eminent organising principle of society, taking precedence over justice and personal rights. With the development of urban civilisation, like the city states and commercial empires of the Greeks and Romans, traditions of public and international law began to evolve, based on the concepts of a rational moral order in Greek philosophy and universal natural justice in Roman law. Though Jewish and early Christian societies incorporated strong elements of beneficent paternalism and concern with social justice, their unique contribution has been to emphasise the demands of an ethic of love—namely, respect for the unique dignity and rights of the individual person. In each of these types of social organisation, where, respectively, beneficence, justice, and respect for persons are the primary organising principles, elements of the other principles can be found.

This is not surprising, for in general social organisation is complex and the moral order must have corresponding complexity or ability to accommodate other principles. Thus in traditional tribal or family life, or in the traditional professions (law, medicine, and the church), the values of beneficent paternalism are paramount but do not necessarily exclude concern with justice for all or respect for certain individual rights. In socialist societies concern with social justice has been paramount, but this does not prevent the socialist state from exercising a kind of paternalistic authority in the name of protective beneficence. While in practice such systems may restrict individual rights and liberties, apologists for socialism would say that without universal social justice individual rights become a luxury enjoyed by the few. Liberal and democratic systems purport to make respect for personal rights and liberty the supreme organising principle of society. But without the built in safeguards of universal justice, or the willingness of the state to act to protect the vulnerable, individuals have no protection against discrimination, injustice, or exploitation by the stronger.

In medicine and the caring professions ethical codes historically have been developed by the professions in response to demands (from the consumer side) that professionals justify the faith clients place in their competence and integrity; but these are also required (from the supply side) to legitimate professional intervention in a crisis. The paradigm for code based ethics is crisis intervention—where the patient is unconscious, incompetent, or extremely vulnerable and the doctor, for example, is required to take action and accept full responsibility for the treatment given. In such a setting the doctor can only fall back on his own personal ethical code or that of his profession. Not surprisingly in code-based ethics protective beneficence, or the duty to care, has paramount importance.

In the consulting professions, where a client voluntarily seeks help with a problem, but is fairly independent, mobile, competent, and continent, and the professional carer is in the position of offering a service, being paid to care, the two parties can be said to enter into a contractual relationship. This contract may be formally negotiated or may be informal and implicit. The crucial difference is that contractual ethics, as distinct from code-based ethics, relates to a setting where the contracting parties recognise mutual and reciprocal rights. Contractual ethics are governed by considerations of justice (including civil and criminal law where necessary).

In situations of chronic or terminal care another kind of model may be required. Because the nature of the therapeutic relationship or pattern of care changes, as do the practical and moral considerations governing both, the "contract" may need to be renegotiated. For example, when a patient is dying, or his condition is chronic, and the doctor has exhausted his repertoire of therapeutic measures, then, assuming that the patient is competent and consultable, to continue to offer care (under the guise of "treatment") would be officious and misleading unless the patient is consulted about the proposed course of palliative care and given the opportunity to accept or reject it. The continuation of the caring relationship under these circumstances requires a different kind of commitment on both sides—what May has called a "covenantal relationship"—because, like a biblical covenant, it requires a commitment of mutual fidelity between the carer and the one cared for. The carer accepts the role of patient advocate and takes on supererogatory duties in return for the love and trust of the patient. In covenantal ethics respect for personal rights takes precedence over considerations of justice or mere beneficence.[26]

Philosophical arguments for the logical priority of certain principles

A philosophical analysis of ethical systems can provide another kind of argument for recognising the existence of certain fundamental ethical principles in health care. The argument is a logical one, based on the formal requirements for a coherent ethical system as such. This type of argument, developed by Immanuel Kant (1724-1804), is descriptive and formal and is not really persuasive or prescriptive unless taken together with the types of arguments already advanced.

In his *Groundwork to the Metaphysic of Morals* (1785) Kant argued that the concept of person or personhood is a primitive concept in ethics.[27] Without it ethics cannot get started, for the concept of person—that is, an individual who is a bearer of rights and responsibilities—is both formally constitutive of ethics and practically definitive of the membership and scope of the moral community.

The concept of person or even a derived list of personal rights, however, would not alone be enough to found a coherent system of ethics. Personal rights or statements of the necessary and sufficient conditons for persons to be persons would not provide an adequate basis for a system of social ethics unless these rights could be justified as rights for all. This requires a principle of universalisability, as Kant called it, which is really a requirement of justice or universal fairness.

Even the concept of persons as bearers of rights and the concept of universal justice, however, would not be sufficient to ensure a workable system of social ethics without a further principle, which might be called the principle of reciprocity—that is, the recognition of a duty to care for others as you would have them care for you. In the real world we are not all equal. At certain times in our lives we are all very vulnerable and unable to claim or defend our rights—as infants, when sick, injured, or mentally disordered, or when senile or dying. Unless we build in a principle of reciprocity we have no way of grounding the obligation to care for the vulnerable. Hence the principles of respect for persons, universal justice, and beneficence mutually imply one another as formal and practical requirements for any coherent system of social ethics.

The purpose of this paper has been to argue the case for recognising certain principles as being fundamental to ethics in general and to medical ethics or the ethics of health care in particular. It is not the purpose of this paper to discuss all their possible practical applications, but a few might be mentioned.

Respect for persons, justice, and beneficence

Respect for persons means basically treating patients as persons—that is, individuals with rights. It means respecting the autonomy of subjects and protecting those who may suffer loss of autonomy through illness, injury, or mental disorder and working to restore autonomy to those who have lost it. It means recognising the fundamental rights of patients as persons—namely, the right to know, the right to privacy, and the right to treatment. Clearly there is a tension among these rights, as in attempting to ensure informed and voluntary consent, in setting sensible limits to confidentiality or physical privacy, or in distinguishing between care and treatment or choices of treatments. Respect for persons means exercising care in such a way as to maintain the optimum level of the patient's autonomy by sharing knowledge and skills as well as treatment with the patient to avoid creating and perpetuating relationships of dependency.

Justice, or the demand for universal fairness, stands in a tense relation with respect for persons. The exercise of individual rights may have to be limited or circumscribed in the interests of the common good—for example, freedom of movement and individual privacy may have to be compromised by public health measures to contain epidemics. We are not concerned here with retributive justice but with distributive justice. There are, however, some analogies with retributive justice in the social controls imposed on the mentally disordered and loss of rights of patients in institutional care, as the sociological analysis of sickness behaviour as a form of deviance shows.[28] [29]

Justice in health care, however, is more broadly concerned with equalising as far as possible the distribution of health care resources and opportunities for care and treatment, tax burdens and responsibilities, and risks and benefits to ensure fairness to individuals and groups. Justice to individuals means primarily non-discrimination on the basis of sex, religion, social standing, political affiliation, youth, old age, handicap, or mental disorder, and equal opportunity in terms of access to resources, including preventive and treatment health services and the benefits of research. Justice in terms of equality of outcome for groups (see, for example, the Black report[30]) relates to the "political" responsibilities and accountability of health workers in controlling and allocating resources and in planning, research, and development. It may also entail accepting responsibility for practising positive discrimination and campaigning for resources as well as maintaining services and defending standards of care and treatment.

Beneficence has tended to enjoy a bad press recently, with much emphasis being given by pressure groups to patients' rights or by politicians to debates about justice and the political economy of health services. Nevertheless, beneficence is an indispensible value in health care, as it is in ethics generally. The duty to care is not only about recognising a reciprocal responsibility for one another but also in particular about recognising a duty to protect the vulnerable—that is, accepting the role of advocate of the rights of those who are unable to defend their own rights. It relates too to the responsibility of health workers to share their knowledge and skill (for "knowledge is power")—that is, to use it to enhance the autonomy, skills, and ability of people to take responsibility for their own lives and their own health, to help themselves to health. This means maximising the educational potential of every clinical encounter and all health workers recognising their need to develop and enhance their education and communication skills.

Conclusion

There are good grounds for us to recognise respect for persons, justice, and beneficence as fundamental principles in ethics—principles with particular meanings and implications when applied to the analysis of relationships between carers and clients in health care (or for that matter to the wider responsibilities of health workers in teaching, research, and planning as well as in the administration of health services). It has not been the purpose of this paper to discuss these practical applications or implications in detail but to set out some of the arguments for the primacy of these principles.

Neither has it been considered appropriate to discuss those second order theories we adduce to justify these principles or any particular rank ordering of them (such as utilitarian, deontological, natural law, or agapistic theories). The basic contention is that respect for persons, justice, and beneficence are fundamental principles in a formal sense. How we view these principles in practice will depend on our particular culture and experience and the kinds of metaethical criteria we use for interpreting, applying, and justifying these principles and others we may derive from them.[31]

1 Bankowski Z, Corvera BJ. *Medical ethics and medical education.* Council for International Organisations of Medical Sciences, 1981.
2 International Council of Nurses. *Code for nurses.* Geneva: International Council of Nurses, 1953.
3 American Nurses' Association. *Code for nurses.* New York: American Nurses' Association, 1968.
4 Royal College of Nursing. *RCN code of professional conduct.* London: Royal College of Nursing, 1976.
5 American Psychological Association. *Ethical principles in the conduct of research with human participants.* New York: APA, 1973.
6 British Association of Social Workers. *Code of ethics for social workers.* London: British Association of Social Workers, 1975.
7 British Association of Social Workers. *Confidentiality in social work.* London: British Association of Social Workers, 1977.

8 Central Council for Education and Training in Social Work. *Values in social work*. London: Central Council for Education and Training in Social Work, 1976.
9 Friedson E. *The profession of medicine*. New York: Dodd, Mead and Co, 1975:23-70.
10 Sigerist HL. On Hippocrates. *Bull Hist Med* 1934;**11**:190-214.
11 Cohn-Haft L. *The public physician of Ancient Greece*. Northampton, Massachusetts: Smith College, 1956.
12 Duncan AS, Dunstan GR, Welbourn RB. *Dictionary of medical ethics*. Revised ed. London: Darton, Longman and Todd, 1981:130-40.
13 United States Department of Health, Education, and Welfare. *Ethical principles and guidelines for the protection of human subjects of research*. Washington, DC: United States Department of Health, Education, and Welfare, 1978. (DHEW publication No 05 78 0012.) (Belmont report.)
14 Friel JP, ed. *Illustrated medical dictionary*. 25th ed. Philadelphia: W B Saunders, 1974.
15 Balint M. *The doctor, his patient and the illness*. Revised ed. London: Pitman Medical, 1974.
16 Gillon R. Beneficence: doing good for others. *Br Med J* 1985;**291**:44-5.
17 Gillon R. "Primus non nocere" and the principle of non-maleficence. *Br Med J* 1985;**291**:130-1.
18 Gillon R. Justice and medical ethics. *Br Med J* 1985;**291**:201-2.
19 Gillon R. Justice and allocation of medical resources. *Br Med J* 1985;**291**:266-8.
20 Gillon R. Telling the truth and medical ethics. *Br Med J* 1985;**291**:1556-8.
21 Gillon R. Confidentiality. *Br Med J* 1985;**291**:1634-6.
22 Gillon R. Consent. *Br Med J* 1985;**291**:1700-1.
23 Gillon R. Where respect for autonomy is not the answer. *Br Med J* 1986;**292**:48-9.
24 Beauchamp T, Childress J. *Principles of bio-medical ethics*. Oxford: Oxford University Press, 1979.
25 Veatch RM. *A theory of medical ethics*. New York: Basic Books, 1981.
26 May W. *Code, covenant, contract or philanthropy?* Hastings-on-Hudson: Hastings Center, 1975.
27 Kant I. (Paton HJ, translator). *The moral law. Groundwork to the metaphysic of morals*. London: Hutchinson University Library, 1785.
28 Cohen AK. *Deviance and control*. New York: Prentice-Hall, 1966.
29 Lemert E. *Social pathology*. New York: McGraw-Hill, 1951.
30 Department of Health and Social Security. *Inequalities in health*. London: DHSS, 1980.
31 Thompson IE. *Nursing ethics*. Edinburgh: Churchill Livingstone, 1983:12543.